T0367129

PICTORIAL ANATOMY OF THE FETAL PIG

PICTORIAL ANATOMY
OF THE
FETAL PIG

Second Edition, Revised and Enlarged

ILLUSTRATIONS AND TEXT BY STEPHEN G. GILBERT

UNIVERSITY OF WASHINGTON PRESS

SEATTLE AND LONDON

First edition copyright © 1963 by the University of
Washington Press
Second edition copyright © 1966 by the University of
Washington Press
Fourth printing with corrections, 1971
Printed in the United States of America

18 17   19 18 17 16

University of Washington Press
www.washington.edu/uwpress

Library of Congress Catalog Card Number 63-10797
ISBN 978-0-295-73877-2

All rights reserved. No part of this publication may be
reproduced or transmitted in any form or by any means,
electronic or mechanical, including photocopy, recording,
or any information storage or retrieval system, without
permission in writing from the publisher.

The paper used in this publication meets the minimum
requirements of American National Standard for Information
Sciences—Permanence of Paper for Printed Library Materials,
ANSI Z39.48-1984. ⊗

Preface

This book was originally designed as a pictorial supplement to be used in connection with other texts. At the request of many teachers, I have expanded the coverage in this edition to include dissecting instructions, descriptive text, and some additional material on the skeleton, muscles, and nervous system. I would like to thank the teachers who were kind enough to write to me, and, as in the past, any suggestions for improving subsequent editions will be welcome. Correspondence should be addressed to me in care of the University of Washington Press.

Acknowledgment is made for special permission to quote the short passage from D'Arcy Wentworth Thompson's *On Growth and Form* (abridged edition, J. T. Bonner, ed.), published by Cambridge University Press, New York; and for the drawing (Fig. 1) from *Three Unpublished Drawings of the Anatomy of the Human Ear* by Max Broedel, published by W. B. Saunders Company, Philadelphia. The illustrations on pages 9, 24, 47, 48, and 51 originally appeared in my *Atlas of General Zoology,* and are reproduced by permission of the publisher, Burgess Publishing Company, Minneapolis, Minn.

I would also like to thank Dr. Richard C. Snyder of the University of Washington, who checked many of the drawings; Miss Bertha B. Hallam of the University of Oregon Medical School Library, who very kindly supplied me with many books and journals; my good friends Arnold Adams, David Barclay, David Stannard, and Ehrick Wheeler, who read and criticized portions of the text; and Al Uberti of the University of Washington Department of Printing, who has been most helpful and patient in solving production problems.

Stephen G. Gilbert

Contents

Introduction

In beginning the study of any subject, it is usually necessary to learn some new words, and your dissection of the fetal pig may be thought of as similar to a vocabulary-building exercise in a foreign language. Essentially, what you will do in this exercise is to connect anatomical names with anatomical structures. This is a necessary first step, but it is *only* a first step and has little value as an end in itself. Naming each part of a fetal pig has no more biological meaning than the recitation of a dictionary has literary meaning. It is what you say with your vocabulary that counts.

I would like to suggest that your exercises in vocabulary building will be more interesting if you think from the beginning in terms of the connection between form and function. You can do this in an elementary way by comparing the pig with the frog, which you have already studied, and attempting to explain the differences between them in functional terms.

Perhaps the most significant difference between the pig and the frog is that the pig is a warm-blooded animal and the frog is a cold-blooded animal. Mammals and birds are warm-blooded, which means that their body temperatures are for the most part intrinsically controlled and remain fairly constant independent of the environmental temperature. All other animals are cold-blooded, which means that their body temperatures usually do not vary more than a few degrees from the temperature of their surroundings.

Almost every time we compare a structure found in the pig with a homologous structure in the frog, we will find a difference which can be interpreted with reference to the development of intrinsic temperature control. The development of the double-pump heart, the elaborate lung structure, the increased length of the alimentary canal, and the adaptations for internal fertilization are a few of the many changes which may be related to this development. The extent to which an animal is capable of intrinsic temperature control also affects its size, its powers of movement, and the range of environmental conditions within which it can survive.

In warm-blooded animals, heat is produced within the body and dissipated through the skin, and thus the direction of heat flow is usually from the animal to the environment. The fur, feathers, and subcutaneous fat of warm-blooded animals serve as insulation to conserve internally produced heat. Reptiles and amphibians draw their body warmth from their surroundings; for them, insulation would be a disadvantage to the extent that it impeded the flow of heat from the environment.

It is perhaps an oversimplification, however, to suppose that insulation could never be an advantage for a cold-blooded animal. There must have been intermediate evolutionary forms in which insulation and intrinsic temperature control were combined to varying extents. A number of living mammals have fur but exhibit only partial temperature control; the bat, marmot, and dwarf mouse are animals which, for various reasons, do not always maintain the high constant body temperatures achieved by most mammals.

An interesting speculation on the origin of fur and feather is given by Raymond B. Cowles, who writes:

> It seems . . . logical to conclude that mutations producing fur and feathers were originally retained because of their function as a device that could retard the absorption rate of excessive solar radiation. Later on, their possession permitted the gradual development of temperature control necessary for the development of warmblooded animals. Without an already acquired insulating coat, it is difficult to understand how energy-expending, internally heated systems could have survived in a cooling environment.

In both warm-blooded and cold-blooded terrestrial vertebrates, the blood plays an important role in equalizing body temperature. The specific heat of water (and therefore of blood, which is 80 per cent water) is higher than that of almost any other substance, and this factor makes blood ideally suited for its role in heat stabilization. In warm-blooded animals, blood absorbs heat in the deep, heat-producing tissues and loses it when passing through the superficial cutaneous vessels, which constrict in cold weather to minimize heat loss. In warm weather, heat loss through the skin is increased by the dilation of the cutaneous vessels and by perspiration.

Vasodilation also occurs in reptiles and amphibians during warm weather. In reptiles, the blood is warmed in the cutaneous vessels and then travels to the deeper parts of the body where its heat is absorbed by the tissues; cooler blood then returns to the skin where it absorbs more heat, and the cycle is repeated. In amphibians, vasodilation facilitates the increased exchange of respiratory gases, which occurs during warm weather, but in them the heat absorption of the blood is minimized because more heat may be lost through evaporation of water from the moist skin than is gained by radiation. Cowles makes this speculation on the role of vasodilation in evolution:

Vascular blood shunting originated in amphibia to serve respiratory needs, was then employed in reptiles to absorb heat, and in the warmbloods to regulate heat. We may assume the probability that these preadaptations in the dermovascular system began to set the stage for vertebrate warmbloodedness in the tetrapods as long ago as possibly the Devonian.

Both warm-blooded and cold-blooded animals strive to operate at optimum temperatures. An animal's method of heat regulation has a great deal to do with the part of the world in which it can operate effectively. If we compare the geographic distribution of warm-blooded animals with that of cold-blooded animals, we find that in general the largest cold-blooded animals live in warm climates. Farther north, the reptiles and amphibians are fewer and smaller than those in the tropics, and north of the Arctic Circle there are only a few species. Among warm-blooded animals, on the other hand, large individuals are successful in both warm and cold climates, and among many forms there is a correlation between low temperature and large body size.

An interesting example of this is provided by the puffins. In Brittany, these birds are but half the size of the puffins native to Spitzbergen. The linear dimensions of the puffins occupying intermediate latitudes increase by over one per cent for each additional degree of north latitude. Similar instances can be found for many warm-blooded forms with relatives in different climates, although, of course, there are exceptions and it should be emphasized that absolute size is only one of many interdependent factors contributing to the success of an animal in a given environment.

The explanation usually given for the difference in distribution between warm-blooded and cold-blooded animals has to do with heat loss and its relation to body surface, and to understand this we must first consider some simple surface-volume relations. In two objects of similar shape but different size, the surface is proportional to the square of the linear dimensions, whereas the volume is proportional to the cube of the linear dimensions. For instance, if we calculate the surfaces and the volumes of two cubes measuring one foot high and ten feet high, we find that in the larger cube the linear dimension has increased by a factor of ten, the surface by a factor of one hundred, and the volume by a factor of one thousand. We see how increases in volume are related to increases in surface by comparing the squares and the cubes of the natural numbers:

1	2	3	4	5	6	7
1	4	9	16	25	36	49
1	8	27	64	125	216	343

In large animals the volume is large compared to the surface; in small animals the volume is small compared to the surface.

The speed with which an animal gains or loses heat depends on the relation between the volume of the animal and the area of skin across which heat transfer occurs. If the area is large in relation to the volume, heat transfer occurs rapidly, but if the area is small in relation to the volume, heat transfer occurs more slowly. Cold-blooded animals can live only in an environment which maintains the body heat within the range necessary for metabolic processes to occur. We do not find the largest cold-blooded terrestrial vertebrates in temperate climates because heat transfer in them occurs slowly due to the relatively small skin area and the available heat is not sufficient to maintain body temperatures at the level required for normal activity. Small cold-blooded animals, on the other hand, do reasonably well in temperate climates because they have a relatively large skin area and a moderate amount of environmental heat will raise their body temperatures to the required level within a reasonable time.

In small warm-blooded animals, heat transfer occurs in the opposite direction. They lose heat rapidly because of their relatively large skin area and therefore do not survive in cold climates unless the food supply is adequate to replace the heat lost by dissipation through the body surface. Large warm-blooded animals lose heat more slowly, and this is one of the factors which makes them successful in cold climates.

An interesting example of heat loss through skin surface is found in the bat, in which much of the body heat is dissipated through the surface of the highly vascular wings. In flight, the bat's body temperature is maintained at a level comparable to that of other warm-blooded animals. While at rest, however, the loss of heat through the uninsulated surface of the wings is apparently so great that the bat is unable to maintain its body temperature, and it becomes virtually cold-blooded. The bat, in fact, practices daily hibernation. Similar temperature reduction is found in other hibernating animals, in which the metabolic rate during hibernation may be 1/20th to 1/100th the normal rate.

Heat loss through a relatively large body surface is one of the reasons why small mammals produce more heat per pound of body weight than large mammals produce. The long-tailed shrew, for instance, loses a great deal of body heat by dissipation through the skin and produces about one hundred times more heat per gram than the cow in order to maintain a comparable body temperature. If a whale produced as much heat per gram as the shrew produces, the temperature of the whale would approach the boiling point.

In cold-blooded animals, too, heat production per gram of body weight is lower in large individuals than it is in small individuals. We do not generally think of cold-blooded animals as producing heat, but calculations show that if a ten-ton shark produced as much heat per unit body weight as the smallest fish (*Schindleria*, 2 mg), its heat production would be four hundred times the actual value. If the shark produced as much heat per unit body weight as the smallest living organisms—bacteria—its heat production would be four thousand times the actual value.

Actually most cold-blooded aquatic vertebrates have body temperatures very slightly above the temperature of the water in which they live and the small amount of heat produced by their low metabolism is almost completely dissipated into the water. In amphibians and reptiles, the temperature balance between the animal and its environment is complicated by the fact that the environmental temperature changes, with the result that the animal alternately gains and loses heat.

Heat production per unit body weight in any animal is affected by body temperature, the size of the animal, and the degree of muscular activity. Comparisons of the heat production of a mammal at rest and of a cold-blooded animal of identical body weight and body temperature show that the heat production of the mammal is approximately five times that of the cold-blooded animal. This relation holds whether the mammal and the cold-blooded animal used for the comparison are small or large. Of course, the variables which are ruled out in this comparison are not ruled out in nature. A frog sitting at the edge of a pond on a typical spring day (weight, 35 grams; body temperature, 16°C) produces only 1/1700 as much heat per unit body weight as a hummingbird in flight (weight, 3.8 grams; body temperature, 41°C).

If a large warm-blooded animal produces a relatively small amount of heat per gram and a small cold-blooded animal produces a relatively large amount of heat per gram, is it possible that a large warm-blooded animal could produce less heat per gram than a small cold-blooded animal? The answer is yes, for a small frog produces about twice as much heat per gram as an elephant produces, yet the frog loses so much heat through its relatively large skin surface that its temperature is very nearly the same as that of its environment, whereas the elephant retains most of its heat and its temperature remains high and constant.

In plants, too, metabolic activity is greater in small individuals than it is in large individuals. A sprouting pea produces more heat per gram than a resting human, and the energy metabolism per unit body weight of the bacteria is attained by the smallest warm-blooded animals during muscular activity.

The fundamental importance of temperature regulation lies in the fact that the chemical processes characteristic of animal life can occur only within a fairly narrow range, from about 0°C (freezing) to somewhat over 40°C. The body temperature of the animals which evolved within the ocean was determined by the aquatic environment. No part of the ocean lies outside the range within which metabolic processes can function, and it is, perhaps, no accident that the temperature range necessary for animal metabolism as we know it coincides with the temperature range of the water within which it evolved.

On land, however, the temperature fluctuates beyond the range within which metabolic processes function. At temperatures lower than about 6°C or higher than about 50°C, most cold-blooded terrestrial animals are inactive. They survive these extremes by such means as hibernation, estivation, encystment, or by laying eggs which will survive temperatures too harsh for the adults.

It may be that the extent of temperature variation is a more important factor than the absolute temperature in limiting animal activity. We reason that alligators cannot survive in cold climates because the available heat is not sufficient to raise their body temperatures to the required level; and yet the giant squid lives in arctic waters at temperatures close to 0°C. If large cold-blooded animals can be active in the ocean at near-freezing temperatures, why can't they be active on land? The answer to this question is not fully understood, but it probably has to do with the difficulty of adapting to temperature change. Apparently it is easier for a cold-blooded animal to adapt to a low constant temperature than to a range of different temperatures.

In addition to maintaining the temperature of an aquatic animal, the water supports much of its weight. A fish can rest motionless with little muscular exertion. When it swims, it does so by alternately contracting the muscles on either side of the body and forcing itself along by the backward pressure of the trunk and tail against the water. A large terrestrial vertebrate, in contrast, must exert considerable muscular force to stand and support the weight of its body, and the energy expended during sustained running on land is many times that required by a rapidly swimming fish. These considerations help to explain the fact that amphibians and reptiles which live in temperate climates move by crawling, as in the case of snakes, lizards, and salamanders, or by hopping, as in the case of frogs and toads. No reptiles exist today that are capable of true flight, and few run with any speed. Apparently the metabolism of modern reptiles and amphibians is too sluggish to sustain such activity. As to the temperature and metabolism of the flying reptiles and the dinosaurs of 150 million years ago, we can only guess.

Biology texts sometimes give the impression that cold-blooded animals always operate at a disadvantage compared to warm-blooded animals. In *The Biology of the Amphibia* Noble writes:

Amphibia are cold-blooded; they lack the mechanisms which give the higher types both freedom from environmental change and constancy of chemical activity at the optimum conditions for the expenditure of their energies. Low body temperature means slow chemical changes, such as those of digestion, also lower velocity of nerve conduction and a throttling down of many other body activities which in the homoiotherms [warm-blooded animals] produce a more active and efficient organism. . . . Amphibia are not able to make use, to the fullest extent, of either their nervous or their motor systems. They remain slaves of their surroundings.

Noble's statement is true in the sense that all the energy-yielding chemical reactions of the frog's metabolism are more sluggish than those of a warm-blooded animal, even when the temperature of the frog is the same as that of the warm-blooded animal. However, the statement is misleading if it leaves one with the impression that a frog would be better off if it were warm-blooded. The adaptive value of intrinsic temperature regulation can be judged only when we consider the animal in relation to its biophysical environment. To see what this means, let us create a warm-blooded frog and test its efficiency against that of an ordinary cold-blooded frog.

The first thing the warm-blooded frog will have to do is maintain its body temperature and metabolism at a high level. Because it has no insulation in the form of fur and subcutaneous fat, the warm-blooded frog will suffer considerably more heat loss than an ordinary mammal of the same size, and in order to maintain its high metabolic rate it will have to eat large quantities of food, especially during winter. But this will present practical difficulties. The frog takes only moving prey; its diet consists of worms, insects, and other small cold-blooded animals which are dormant during the winter. Frogs are

inactive in cold weather for the same reason as insects and other small invertebrates: their metabolism slows down, resulting in minimal requirements for food and oxygen. Frogs can live for many months without food, and some amphibians have survived fasts of over a year.

For protection in cold weather, frogs often hibernate in water which is near the freezing point. The low temperature of the water reduces the frog's metabolic rate and therefore it needs little oxygen. This, together with the fact that cold water contains more dissolved oxygen than warm water, enables the frog to survive without using its lungs, because the exchange of oxygen and carbon dioxide which occurs between the frog's skin and the water is adequate for its needs.

What would happen if our imaginary warm-blooded frog were to spend the winter in cold water? It is a relatively small animal with a surface large in proportion to its volume; therefore, it will lose heat rapidly, and of course it will lose heat even more rapidly in cold water than in air of the same temperature. The heat loss will be so great, in fact, that no matter how much food it consumes it will not be able to maintain its body temperature in water near the freezing point. No warm-blooded animal the size of a frog could survive very long in such water; for this we shall need a whale.

Perhaps we can get around this problem by providing our frog with a fur coat and a layer of subcutaneous fat so that it can hibernate like a bear. If we do this, however, we will find that the frog can no longer absorb water through its skin by osmosis (which is its only means of water intake) and that it can no longer employ cutaneous respiration, which accounts for about 50 per cent of its exchange of oxygen and carbon dioxide with the atmosphere.

These difficulties present examples of the fact that it is impossible to take an isolated biological feature and discuss its advantages or disadvantages out of context. The frog's mechanisms of temperature control, metabolism, and respiration are an integral part of its structure and way of life. None of these features can be changed without affecting the others. In creating a warm-blooded frog, we found that we no longer had a frog at all. In fact, something like this happened when the first reptiles (not frogs) began to develop intrinsic temperature control. They were on their way to evolving into mammals.

In many cases, the low metabolism of cold-blooded animals can be a definite advantage, as it was, for instance, in the case of the first vertebrates which adopted a partially terrestrial life. Some idea of their habits can be gained from their relative, the modern lungfish, which breathes by means of lungs instead of gills. In the water its habits are much like those of other fish, except that it rises to the surface every ten or fifteen minutes for a breath of air. The lungfish inhabits shallow waters which occasionally dry up and leave it stranded. When this happens, it digs a burrow in the mud and retires to wait for the water to rise again. Lungfish have lived for four years without food in captivity, and it is estimated that they can survive fasts of up to seven years under natural conditions.

The adaptive value of the lungfish's ability to live without food is related to its evolution in an environment where both food and water were sometimes scarce. The invasion of the land by life from the water was a slow process. Plants gradually emerged and established themselves on land, to be followed by small invertebrate forms. The first vertebrates, which probably ventured out of the water in search of small invertebrate prey, were invading a world in which the sphere of life as we know it today did not exist. The low metabolism of these cold-blooded vertebrates enabled them to survive under conditions which would have been impossible for a warm-blooded animal with its constant need for food.

Only after vertebrates had been established on land for about 150 million years did intrinsic temperature control begin to develop. "The basic placental mammal," writes George Gaylord Simpson, "occupied a particular niche in the ecology of its time. It was an active, tiny, quadrupedal type of animal, with its obscurity as main defense, eating mainly small animal food such as worms or insects and their larva." For about 100 million years, then, primitive mammals occupied a relatively inconspicuous place in a world dominated by giant reptiles. Modern mammalian forms did not begin to develop until about 70 million years ago, after most of the giant reptiles had become extinct. This illustrates the point that the advantages of intrinsic temperature control depend on the kind of competition an animal faces and on the environment in which it lives. Mammals living in a tropical environment dominated by reptiles never evolved beyond the basic form described by Simpson.

Many modern amphibians and reptiles are relatively recent evolutionary developments which have become adapted to the same ecological niche occupied for so long by primitive mammals. The tables are turned, and now in many cases it is the reptile and the amphibian which depend on obscurity for their defense and live on worms, insects, and grubs, playing a minor role in a world dominated by mammals.

The evolution of intrinsic temperature control is one of the many examples of the fact that evolution follows lines determined by the functional interrelationship between the animal and its biophysical environment, and that each individual is very literally an integral part of that environment.

We are so accustomed to speaking of biological form as opposed to function that we are apt to think that we are talking about two different things when we use these words. In reality we are referring to different aspects of a single phenomenon. Each individual animal grows and functions according to genetically coded plans which develop and are transmitted and modified over millions of generations. These plans may be thought of as an organized system of molecules which are constantly in exchange with the molecules of the environment. We study this molecular exchange as "metabolism." When this form of exchange ceases, another pattern of exchange can be recognized and the organization of molecules which we identified as an individual is broken down by the actions of plants and animals into compounds which are re-exchanged with other systems.

You should remember, therefore, that your fetal pig preserved in formalin is an artifact made by man. It is an artificially arrested stage in a process with connections which might be traced indefinitely in space and time, and it is in tracing these connections that your study of anatomy will become meaningful and interesting.

PICTORIAL
ANATOMY
OF THE
FETAL PIG

THE SKELETON

Bone is composed of two different kinds of tissue: *compact* and *cancellous*. Compact bone always forms the exterior, whereas cancellous bone is always found in the interior. These two kinds of bone are variously combined to provide optimum strength with a minimum of material.

A fibrous membrane, the *periosteum*, covers the surface of each bone, being absent only at the cartilaginous extremities. The cavities of the bones are filled with *marrow*. In youth only red marrow (a blood-forming substance) is found, but in adults much of this is replaced by yellow marrow, which is similar to fat. Each bone is supplied by arteries, veins, nerves, and lymphatics which pass through the compact bone to reach the marrow.

Bones are united by the following types of joints:

1. Immovable *(synarthroses)*. Example: the sutures of the skull, in which the bones are held together by interlocking margins united by fibrous tissue.

2. Movable *(diarthroses)*. Example: the knee, in which the opposing ends of the bones are covered by articular cartilage and held together by ligaments. This type includes most of the joints.

3. Slightly movable *(amphiarthroses)*. Example: the pubic symphysis, in which the bones are held together by a flattened disc of fibrocartilage.

The skeleton of the fetal pig is unsuitable for classroom study because of its immature condition, and the skeleton of the cat will be used instead. Although the proportions of the pig and cat skeletons are different, the bones are homologous and the origins and insertions of the muscles described in the fetal pig may be traced on the cat skeleton. An illustration of the fetal pig skeleton is included for reference. Study the articulated and disarticulated cat skeletons and familiarize yourself with the names of the bones illustrated.

Look at the *femur* of the disarticulated cat skeleton. On the posterior side near the proximal and distal articular surfaces, you will find the *nutrient foramina* which admit vessels and nerves to the medullary cavity. Similar foramina may be found in many other bones.

If your cat skeleton was made from a relatively young animal, you will see *epiphysial lines* between the ends of the femur and the shaft. Similar lines will be seen in the other long bones of the limbs. The epiphysial lines represent the junction between the centers of ossification in the ends *(epiphyses)* and the shaft *(diaphysis)* of the bone. In the illustration of the fetal pig skeleton, you will see that the ends of the femur still consist of unossified cartilage. Soon after birth, centers of ossification appear in the epiphyses. In the young animal, growth occurs at the cartilaginous joint between the diaphysis and the epiphysis, and at maturity the epiphysis becomes fully ossified and fuses with the diaphysis.

The wired and mounted skeleton as seen in a commercial preparation consists only of the inorganic or mineral portion of the bone. Gone are the periosteum, ligaments, nerves, vessels, and organic constituents which form an integral part of the bone in life. D'Arcy Wentworth Thompson describes the difference between the mounted skeleton and the living skeleton as follows:

The "skeleton" as we see it in a museum is a poor and even a misleading picture of mechanical efficiency. From the engineer's point of view, it is a diagram showing all the compression-lines, but by no means all of the tension-lines of the construction; it shows all the struts, but few of the ties, and perhaps we might even say *none* of the principal ones; it falls all to pieces unless we clamp it together, as best we can, in a more or less clumsy and immobilized way. But in life, that fabric of struts is surrounded and interwoven with a complicated system of ties—"its living mantles jointed strong, with glistering band and silvery thong": ligament and membrane, muscle and tendon, run between bone and bone; and the beauty and strength of the mechanical construction lie not in one part or in another, but in the harmonious concatenation which all the parts, soft and hard, rigid and flexible, tension-bearing and pressure-bearing, make up together.

Both the external and internal architecture of the bones are subject to modifications due to stresses imposed by life. Cancellous bone, for instance, is constantly renewed. If a broken bone heals so that new stresses are formed, the cancellous bone realigns itself along new structural patterns. Stress can also act as a stimulus to growth itself. If most of the central shaft of the tibia is surgically removed in a young dog, the stimulus of the additional

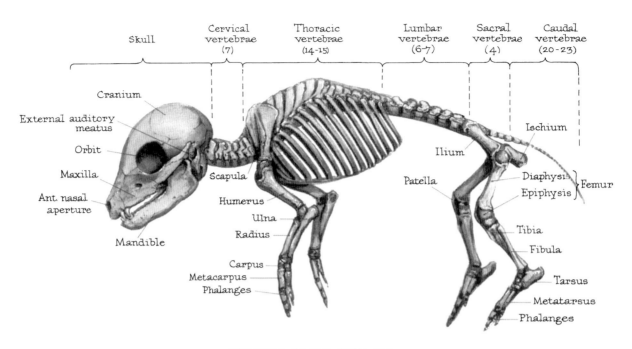

Skull
Cervical vertebrae (7)
Thoracic vertebrae (14-15)
Lumbar vertebrae (6-7)
Sacral vertebrae (4)
Caudal vertebrae (20-23)

Cranium
External auditory meatus
Orbit
Maxilla
Ant. nasal aperture
Mandible
Scapula
Humerus
Ulna
Radius
Carpus
Metacarpus
Phalanges

Ilium
Patella
Ischium
Diaphysis
Epiphysis
Femur
Tibia
Fibula
Tarsus
Metatarsus
Phalanges

SKELETON OF THE FETAL PIG

weight on the fibula will cause the fibula to replace the tibia in size and strength.

Living bone can be transplanted from one part of the body to another. If a fragment is taken from the shaft of a long bone, stripped of periosteum and marrow, and grafted into a muscle or under the skin, the graft will be progressively and completely absorbed by the surrounding tissue, and new bone will grow in the place from which the graft was taken. Bone may be grown in cultures outside the body. When this is done, the bone cells migrate into the culture medium and form systems of bony bars and cartilage. Human bone can be repaired by grafts of processed bone from calves. Several months after the operation the graft is assimilated so completely that it is indistinguishable from the human bone.

Unlike many other structural materials, bone stands up about as well under compression as it does under tension. Because of the variety of stresses to which the body is subjected, its frame must be able to withstand both compression and tension equally well. This is a condition which would disqualify many materials. Granite, for instance, is heavier than bone, does not withstand as much compression as bone, and will break under tension at one-fifteenth the weight which bone supports. White oak weighs less than half as much as bone and supports almost as much weight under tension, but under compression it breaks at less than one-third the weight which bone will

support. To find a substance with qualities comparable to those of bone we must go to medium steel. It weighs four times as much as bone, but withstands about four times as much tension and four times as much compression. A skeleton made of hollow steel rods would be smaller in total volume, but about equal in weight and strength, to a skeleton made of bone.

In structure as well as composition, bone exhibits many adaptations to its role in the economy of the body. An instance of such adaptation is found in the relation of the diameter of the bone to the total weight of the animal. The strength of a shaft is proportional to the area of its cross section (or to the square of its linear dimensions), whereas the weight of a shaft is proportional to the cube of its linear dimensions. Therefore a medium-sized tree will make a bridge across a stream, but for a very long bridge a very large tree of similar proportions will not do because it breaks under its own weight. The bones of the lion are relatively thicker than those of the cat, and the elephant has such heavy bones that it spends considerable effort carrying the bones which support the muscles. For this reason the elephant does not run as the deer. In large aquatic animals, on the other hand, such disproportionate increase in the size of the bones does not occur because the weight of the body is supported directly by the water instead of being transmitted to the ground by legs.

SKELETON OF THE CAT

Cranium
Orbit
Zygomatic arch
Atlas
Axis
Spine of 7th cervical vertebra
Scapular spine
Coracoid
Greater tuberosity
Head of humerus in glenoid fossa
Scapula
Acromion
Sternum
Medial epicondyle of humerus
Olecranon
Humerus
Lateral epicondyle of humerus
Head of radius
Radius
Ulna
Carpus
Metacarpus
Phalanges
Medial malleolus
Costal cartilage
13 thoracic vertebra
Intervertebral foramen
7 th lumbar vertebra
Iliac crest
Ilium
Sacrum
Pubis
Lesser trochanter
Pubic symphysis
Obturator foramen
Medial epicondyle
Head of femur in acetabulum
Greater trochanter
Ischium
Ischiac tuberosity
Femur
Lateral epicondyle of femur
Lateral condyle of tibia
Fibula
Tibia
Patella
Ant. tibial crest
Caudal vertebra
Calcaneus
Tarsus
Lateral malleolus
Metatarsus
Phalanges

5

In small terrestrial animals, total weight is not such an important factor in determining the diameter of the bones. The bones of the deer are not disproportionately thick compared with those of the mouse, even though the deer outweighs the mouse by a factor of several thousand. The femur of the cat is relatively greater in diameter than the femur of man, and yet the human femur carries a disproportionately heavy load. The weight of the animal is only one of several interdependent variables which affect the diameter of the bones. Other variables are the internal architecture of the bone, the strength of the compact bony tissue, and the surface required for muscle attachment.

An example of mechanical adaptation is found in the elbow and the ankle, which are equipped with levers in the form of the *olecranon* and the *calcaneus*. Why is there no such lever at the knee? It is apparent that the arrangement at the elbow and the ankle provides more efficient leverage than the arrangement at the knee, where the tendon of the *quadriceps femoris*, the large extensor of the leg, passes around the joint to insert on the tibia. The answer to this question apparently lies in the fact that considerable weight is transferred directly from bone to bone at the knee (hence the large articular surfaces), but not at the ankle or the elbow, where the joints bend in the other direction and the weight must be sustained by muscle and tendon. In the case of the Achilles tendon, the tensile strain may be considerable, as is demonstrated by the fact that in man it sometimes ruptures during violent exertion.

In the frog, there is no lever at the ankle; the tendon of the gastrocnemius passes around the joint and inserts on the fascia of the foot. In larger animals, such as the lion, cow, and horse, the olecranon and calcaneus are relatively longer than they are in the cat. In the frog, the weight of the body is apparently insufficient to make a lever at the ankle necessary. In the cat, a short lever is required; and in larger animals, a longer lever compensates for the disproportionate increase in weight.

Bone exhibits many internal as well as external structural adaptations. The internal structure of bone may be illustrated by a longitudinal section of the cat's femur. The cylindrical shape of the shaft is an adaptation which enables the bone to resist stresses in any direction. If the shaft were hollow but elliptical in cross section, it would be stronger in the direction of the major axis than in the direction of the minor axis; if the same amount of bone formed a narrow, solid tube, it would be much weaker. The expanded distal end of the femur provides an economical distribution of weight on the articular surface. Like most weight-carrying bones, the femur contains cancellous bone which forms slender spicules or trabeculae at the proximal and distal ends of the shaft. These trabeculae convey the weight from the articular surfaces to the shaft. Trabeculae are not found in the middle of the bone because here all the weight is supported by the walls of the shaft. In a short bone, such as the body of a vertebra, on the other hand, there is no central cavity and we find parallel trabecular columns throughout.

Comparing the femur of the human with that of the cat, we find structural adaptations connected with the increased weight which the human femur carries. The walls of the shaft are much thicker toward the middle, a reflection of the fact that in a bending shaft the stress is greatest at the midpoint. Another adaptation to the increased load is found in the trabecular systems, which follow lines of tension and compression formed as a result of the stresses to which the bone is subjected. In the cat, the load is relatively light and these trabecular systems are not clearly defined.

The skeleton of the bird provides another interesting example of internal structural adaptation. The bones of the wing are not weight-carrying bones; no thickening at the middle of the shaft and no expansion of the articular surfaces occurs in them. Instead of a trabecular system for conveying stress from the articular surface to the shaft, in the largest soaring birds we find the development of diagonal elements which stiffen the bone in a manner similar to the bracing used in the main ribs of airplane wings.

Many other examples of mechanical adaptation can be found throughout the skeleton. Compare the mounted skeletons of the frog and the cat with reference to their adaptation for different modes of life. If cut sections of bones from birds and mammals are available, compare them in terms of structural efficiency.

An excellent introduction to the study of the skeleton can be found in chapter 16, "On Form and Mechanical Efficiency," of D'Arcy Wentworth Thompson's masterpiece, *On Growth and Form*, from which many of the examples in this chapter were borrowed.

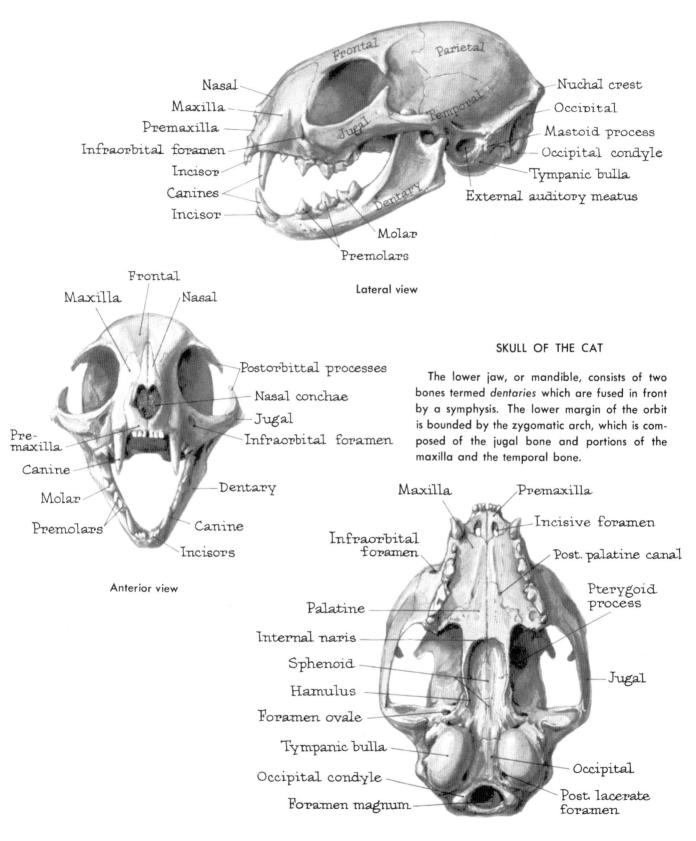

Nasal

Maxilla

Premaxilla

Infraorbital foramen

Incisor

Canines

Incisor

Frontal

Parietal

Temporal

Jugal

Dentary

Molar

Premolars

Nuchal crest

Occipital

Mastoid process

Occipital condyle

Tympanic bulla

External auditory meatus

Lateral view

Frontal

Maxilla

Nasal

Postorbittal processes

Nasal conchae

Jugal

Infraorbital foramen

Pre-maxilla

Canine

Molar

Premolars

Dentary

Canine

Incisors

Anterior view

SKULL OF THE CAT

The lower jaw, or mandible, consists of two bones termed *dentaries* which are fused in front by a symphysis. The lower margin of the orbit is bounded by the zygomatic arch, which is composed of the jugal bone and portions of the maxilla and the temporal bone.

Maxilla

Premaxilla

Incisive foramen

Infraorbital foramen

Post. palatine canal

Pterygoid process

Palatine

Internal naris

Sphenoid

Hamulus

Foramen ovale

Tympanic bulla

Occipital condyle

Foramen magnum

Jugal

Occipital

Post. lacerate foramen

Inferior view

7

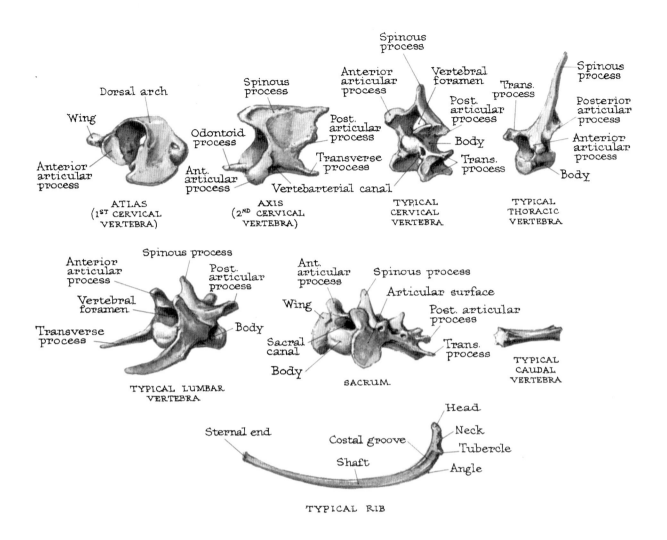

ATLAS
(1ST CERVICAL
VERTEBRA)

AXIS
(2ND CERVICAL
VERTEBRA)

TYPICAL
CERVICAL
VERTEBRA

TYPICAL
THORACIC
VERTEBRA

TYPICAL LUMBAR
VERTEBRA

SACRUM

TYPICAL
CAUDAL
VERTEBRA

TYPICAL RIB

VERTEBRAE OF THE CAT

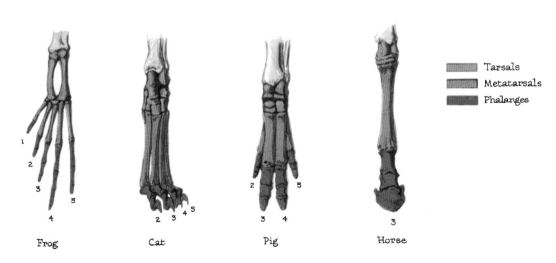

Tarsals
Metatarsals
Phalanges

Frog

Cat

Pig

Horse

HOMOLOGOUS BONES IN THE LEFT HIND FEET OF THE
FROG, CAT, PIG, AND HORSE

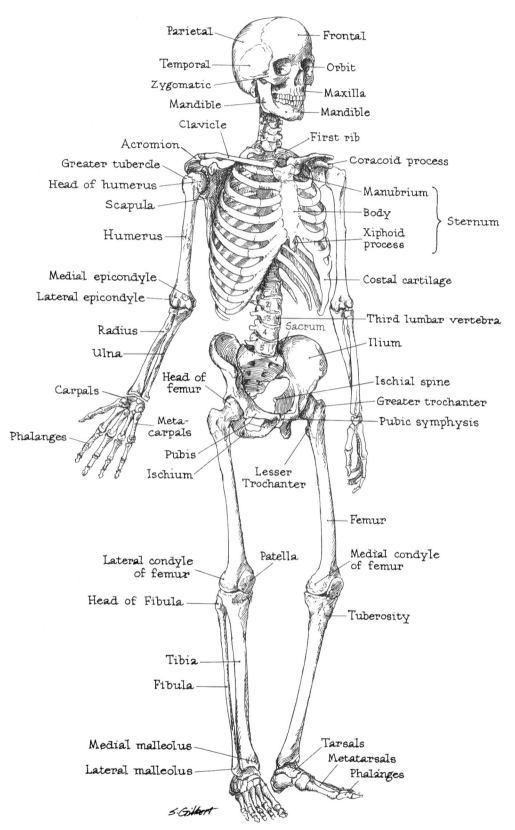

Parietal

Frontal

Temporal

Orbit

Zygomatic

Maxilla

Mandible

Mandible

Clavicle

First rib

Acromion

Coracoid process

Greater tubercle

Head of humerus

Manubrium

Scapula

Body

Sternum

Humerus

Xiphoid
process

Medial epicondyle

Costal cartilage

Lateral epicondyle

Third lumbar vertebra

Radius

Sacrum

Ilium

Ulna

Head of
femur

Ischial spine

Carpals

Greater trochanter

Meta-
carpals

Pubic symphysis

Phalanges

Pubis

Ischium

Lesser
Trochanter

Femur

Lateral condyle
of femur

Patella

Medial condyle
of femur

Head of Fibula

Tuberosity

Tibia

Fibula

Medial malleolus

Tarsals
Metatarsals
Phalanges

Lateral malleolus

S. Gilbert

HUMAN SKELETON, VENTROLATERAL VIEW

THE MUSCLES

No two systems are more closely related in form and function than the muscles and the skeleton. The shapes of the bones are meaningless considered apart from the leverage they provide for the muscles, and the attachments of the muscles can be understood only with reference to the skeleton. Study the bones and the muscles as a single functional unit and refer frequently to the skeleton during your dissection of the muscles.

The fleshy central portion of a skeletal or voluntary muscle consists of contractile muscle fibers and is termed the *belly*. It is usually attached at both ends by connective tissue fibers which form either a tendon or a flat sheet termed an *aponeurosis*, although in some cases muscle fibers attach directly to the periosteum without the intervention of a tendon. The more stable of the two attachments is the *origin*; the more mobile attachment is the *insertion*. The origin is usually nearer the sagittal plane than the insertion. In certain cases a muscle may have more than one belly, and more than one muscle may attach by a common tendon.

Most muscles are attached to bones, cartilages, or ligaments. Muscles may also attach to the fascia covering another muscle, to the mucous membrane (tongue muscles), to the skin (facial muscles), or they may form circular bands (sphincters).

Muscles act only by contraction and almost always occur in antagonistic groups. Examples of such groups are: *extensors*, which straighten joints, and *flexors*, which bend them; *adductors*, which move appendages toward the median plane, and *abductors*, which move them away; *pronators*, which turn the dorsal surface of a limb anteriorly, and *supinators*, which turn the ventral surface of a limb anteriorly; *levators*, which raise structures, and *depressors*, which lower them; *sphincters*, which close openings, and *dilators*, which open them.

Although each muscle is an independent unit in the sense that it has its own arterial, venous, lymphatic, and nervous supply, a muscle rarely acts alone. Almost all bodily movements are the result of the coordinated actions of many muscles. An individual muscle, therefore, may perform a variety of different actions depending on the state of contraction of the other muscles which work with it and against it.

For descriptive purposes we usually speak of a muscle as having a *primary action*, determined by the origin and insertion, and a number of *secondary actions*, determined by the activities of other muscles. In the brief descriptions given in this chapter, only the primary action of each muscle is listed, and in many cases the account of the origin and insertion is considerably abbreviated. In a survey of this scope, the inclusion of every muscle is, of course, impractical; the muscles described have been chosen because they are relatively easy to identify in the fetal pig and because they illustrate the general principles of muscular action.

In the neck of your specimen, you will find an incision through which latex was injected into one of the jugular veins. Make your lateral dissection of the muscles on the side opposite this incision, as the neck muscles will be damaged in the area where the injection was made. Using scissors and being careful to cut only through the skin, make a small V-shaped cut in the shoulder region. Grasp the point of the V with forceps and pull the skin away from the body, using the dull edge of your scalpel to separate the skin from the muscles and connective tissue. Continue in this manner, removing small areas of skin at a time, until you have skinned the entire dorsal and lateral aspects of the trunk, head, and limbs. As you do this, notice the thin muscle fibers which seem to be attached directly to the skin in the area of the face, neck, shoulders, and trunk. These are fibers of the *cutaneus*, a thin, superficial muscular layer which has very little attachment to the skeleton. The contraction of the cutaneus causes the skin to twitch, getting rid of insects and other irritants.

After skinning your specimen, you should identify the salivary glands, which will be removed during the study of the neck muscles. To do this, turn to page 18 and follow the directions on that page. After identifying the

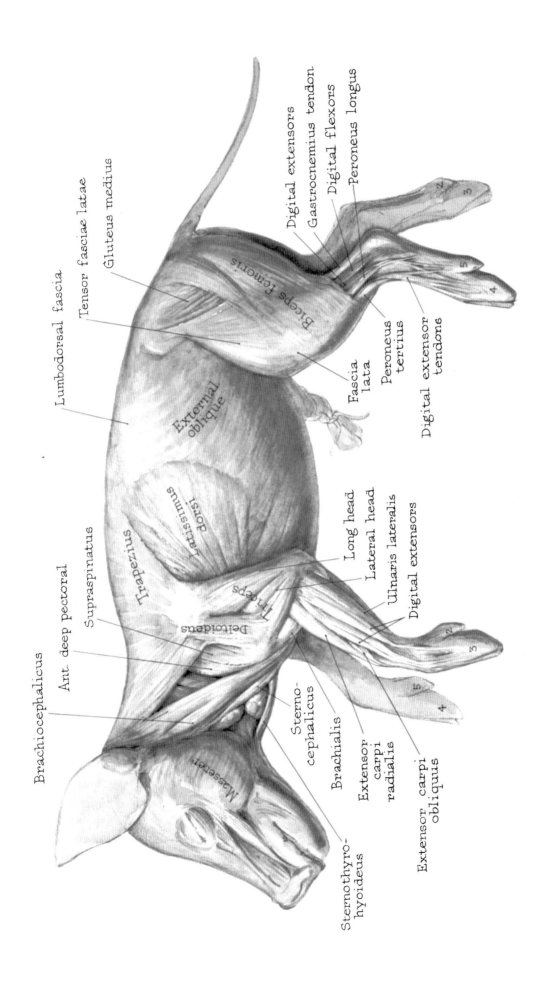

Brachiocephalicus

Ant. deep pectoral

Supraspinatus

Trapezius

Latissimus dorsi

Deltoideus

Triceps

Sternothyro-hyoideus

Sternocephalicus

Brachialis

Extensor carpi radialis

Extensor carpi obliquus

Masseter

Long head

Lateral head

Ulnaris lateralis

Digital extensors

Lumbodorsal fascia

Tensor fasciae latae

Gluteus medius

Biceps femoris

External oblique

Fascia lata

Peroneus tertius

Digital extensor tendons

Digital extensors

Gastrocnemius tendon

Digital flexors

Peroneus longus

MUSCLES OF THE FETAL PIG, LATERAL VIEW

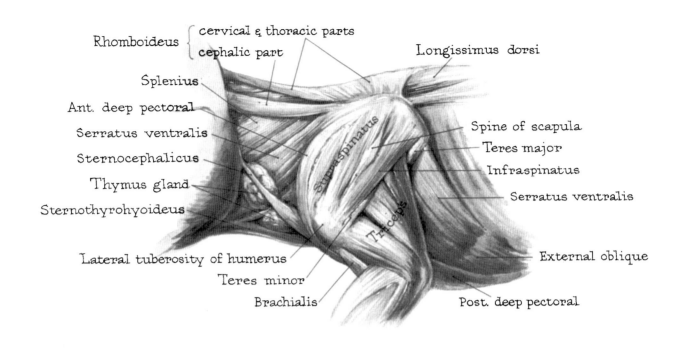

Rhomboideus {cervical & thoracic parts / cephalic part

Splenius

Ant. deep pectoral

Serratus ventralis

Sternocephalicus

Thymus gland

Sternothyrohyoideus

Lateral tuberosity of humerus

Teres minor

Brachialis

Longissimus dorsi

Supraspinatus

Triceps

Spine of scapula

Teres major

Infraspinatus

Serratus ventralis

External oblique

Post. deep pectoral

MUSCLES OF THE SHOULDER, LATERAL VIEW

salivary glands, remove them together with the facial and internal maxillary veins.

After your specimen is skinned, the muscles will not appear as clearly defined as they are in the illustrations. This is because they are covered by loose connective tissue and fat. In addition, each muscle is enclosed within a closely fitting fascial sheath which serves to separate it from the surrounding muscles and maintain it in its proper position relative to them. In some cases, you will find that the boundaries of a muscle are readily apparent, but in other cases a muscle will seem to blend with those around it. This is particularly true of the *trapezius, latissimus dorsi, deltoideus, biceps femoris,* and *tensor fasciae latae.* In order to define the limits of a muscle, use small scissors and forceps to trim away the overlying fat, connective tissue and fascia until you can see the direction of the muscle fibers. Look for a change in the direction of the fibers near the place where the edge of the muscle should be, and attempt to slip the flat edge of your scalpel handle between two separate layers of muscle at this point. If one layer separates readily from another, you have your scalpel handle between two different muscles. Do not try to cut or force the separation of the muscles; if you are looking in the right place, the separation will

be natural. Now identify the muscles illustrated on page 11. The origins, insertions, and actions of the muscles are listed alphabetically on pages 16 and 17.

Cut the *deltoideus* and trim it away completely at both origin and insertion to reveal the *infraspinatus,* which lies beneath it. Be careful not to confuse these two muscles. The deltoideus in the fetal pig is very thin and is attached superficially to the aponeurosis covering the infraspinatus and to the fascia of the limb. The infraspinatus is much thicker than the deltoideus and originates directly from the scapula.

Now identify the *supraspinatus.* Near its insertion, the supraspinatus divides into two branches. One branch inserts on the lateral side of the humerus and the other branch inserts on the anterior side of the humerus. Do not mistake the division between these two branches for the line of separation between the supraspinatus and the infraspinatus. The supraspinatus lies anterior to the spine of the scapula; the infraspinatus lies posterior to the spine.

Cut the *brachiocephalicus* at the origins on the mastoid process and the nuchal crest. Free it from the underlying muscles but do not cut its insertion near the humerus where it seems to blend with the *anterior deep pectoral.* Cut

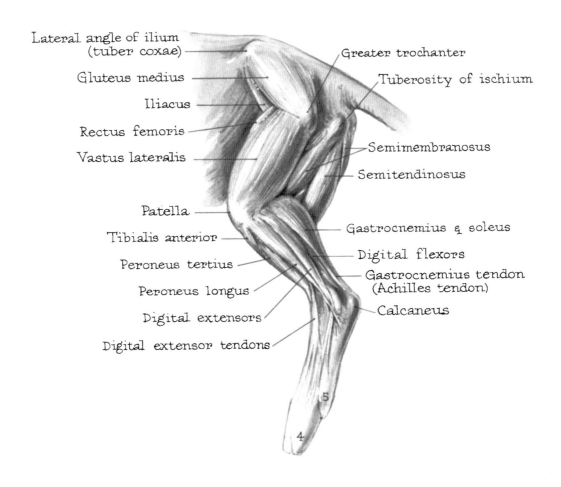

Lateral angle of ilium (tuber coxae)

Gluteus medius

Iliacus

Rectus femoris

Vastus lateralis

Patella

Tibialis anterior

Peroneus tertius

Peroneus longus

Digital extensors

Digital extensor tendons

Greater trochanter

Tuberosity of ischium

Semimembranosus

Semitendinosus

Gastrocnemius & soleus

Digital flexors

Gastrocnemius tendon (Achilles tendon)

Calcaneus

MUSCLES OF THE HINDLIMB, LATERAL VIEW

the trapezius at its insertion on the spine of the scapula. Separate it from the underlying muscles, leaving its origin intact. Be careful not to cut the fibers of the *rhomboideus* which lie parallel to and just below those of the trapezius. Distinguish these two muscles by observing that the fibers of the rhomboideus go directly to the medial border of the scapula, whereas those of the trapezius go to the spine of the scapula.

Cut the *latissimus dorsi* at its origin and trim away the major portion of this muscle, leaving about an inch at the insertion. To establish the origin of the *serratus ventralis,* insert the flat edge of your scalpel handle beneath the scapula and move it ventrally between the serratus ventralis and the thorax.

You were instructed to leave the attachments of certain muscles uncut because it is sometimes difficult to establish the relations of the deep and superficial layers after the superficial muscles are removed. After identifying the muscles illustrated above, you may trim away the remaining portions of the superficial muscles in order to make a neat dissection.

Free the tensor *fasciae latae* along its lateral border and its insertion, but leave the medial portion and the origin intact. Cut the insertion of the *biceps femoris* near the tibia, and peel the aponeurosis back from the leg to expose the muscles of the leg and foot. Lift the biceps femoris, freeing it from the underlying muscles, but leave the origin intact. Below it find branches of the *obturator* and *posterior femoral* arteries together with the *sciatic* nerve and its branches, lying between the *vastus lateralis* in front and the *semitendinosus* behind. Remove these nerves and vessels to identify the *semimembranosus*, which lies beneath them. Identify the other muscles illustrated above.

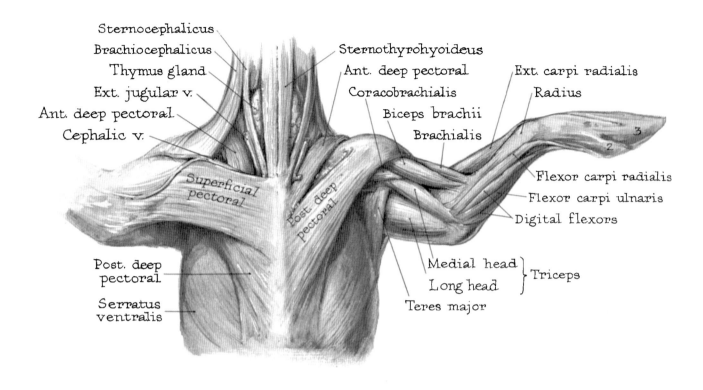

Sternocephalicus
Brachiocephalicus
Thymus gland
Ext. jugular v.
Ant. deep pectoral
Cephalic v.
Superficial pectoral
Post. deep pectoral
Post. deep pectoral
Serratus ventralis

Sternothyrohyoideus
Ant. deep pectoral
Coracobrachialis
Biceps brachii
Brachialis

Ext. carpi radialis
Radius
Flexor carpi radialis
Flexor carpi ulnaris
Digital flexors
Medial head ⎫ Triceps
Long head ⎭
Teres major

MUSCLES OF THE VENTRAL THORACIC REGION

(Right side: superficial muscles. Left side: deep muscles)

To dissect the muscles from the ventral aspect, tie a string around the forefeet of your specimen, pass the string around the back of the dissecting pan, and tie it to the opposite forefoot so that the forelimbs are stretched out at right angles to the body. Do the same with the hindlimbs. Make a midventral incision through the skin from the jaw to the anus. Cut around the umbilical cord and leave it intact. Then make incisions along the ventral sides of the forelimbs and hindlimbs and skin the ventral aspect of your specimen.

You will probably find it convenient to make your deep dissection of the muscles on the same side on which you made the lateral dissection. Leave all the muscles, nerves, and vessels intact on the other side so they can be traced when the circulatory and nervous systems are studied.

The specimen illustrated on the opposite page is a female. If your specimen is a male you will find the penis and the scrotal sacs near the midline behind the umbilical cord. These structures lie between the skin and the superficial muscles, and it will be necessary to move them to one side in order to examine the underlying muscles. Be care-

ful, however, not to cut or damage them. See the penis and scrotal sacs as illustrated on pages 23 and 24.

Slip the flat end of your scalpel between the superficial pectoral (which is very thin) and the posterior deep pectoral muscles to establish the separation between them. Then cut the belly of the superficial pectoral muscle across the midline and trim it away at both the origin and the insertion, removing the cephalic vein at the same time. Find the brachial vessels and branches of the brachial plexus of nerves lying beneath the posterior deep pectoral muscle and extending from its lateral border to the elbow. Cut these structures on one side to reveal the underlying muscles. Identify the insertion of the latissimus dorsi, which was cut during the lateral dissection of the shoulder muscles. Observe that it lies between the teres major and the triceps and inserts on the medial side of the humerus in common with the teres major. Then trim away the insertions of the latissimus dorsi to see the relations of the teres major and the triceps. Remove the connective tissue, fat, and fascia from the forelimb and identify the other muscles illustrated above.

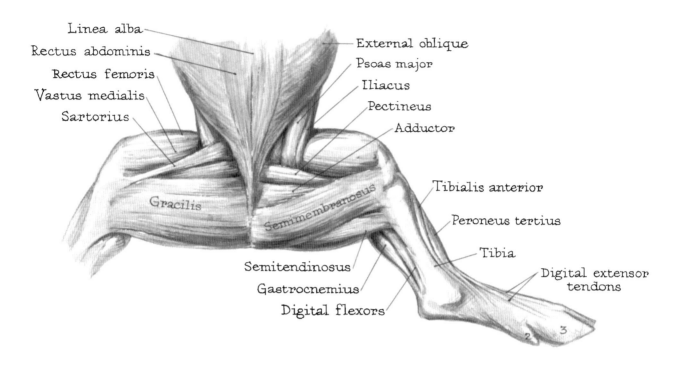

Linea alba
Rectus abdominis
Rectus femoris
Vastus medialis
Sartorius
Gracilis
External oblique
Psoas major
Iliacus
Pectineus
Adductor
Semimembranosus
Tibialis anterior
Peroneus tertius
Tibia
Digital extensor tendons
Semitendinosus
Gastrocnemius
Digital flexors

MUSCLES OF THE HINDLIMB, VENTRAL VIEW
(Right side: superficial muscles. Left side: deep muscles)

Insert your scalpel handle between the *gracilis* and the *sartorius* and separate them from the *pectineus*, *adductor*, and *semimembranosus*, which lie below them. Note that the sartorius and the gracilis are very thin and that their fibers run in almost the same direction as the fibers of the muscles below them. Cut the gracilis and sartorius near their insertions, leaving the origins intact, and peel them back. Under the sartorius you will find the *femoral* vessels. Remove them to expose the underlying muscles.

The term *quadriceps femoris* is applied to the large mass of muscle which covers the anterior surface of the femur and acts as the extensor of the leg. It consists of four muscles which insert by a common tendon on the patella and the tibia: the *rectus femoris*, the *vastus lateralis*, the *vastus medialis*, and the *vastus intermedius*. The vastus intermedius lies deep to the preceding muscles and is not illustrated.

The lateral abdominal wall consists of three muscles: the *external oblique* (the most superficial), the *internal oblique* (the middle layer) and the *transversus* (the deepest layer). These three muscles insert by fascial sheets which pass around the *rectus abdominus* to form a strong aponeurotic covering termed the *rectus sheath*. The anterior and posterior sides of this sheath fuse in the midline, making a tendinous band which extends from the pubis to the sternum. This band is the *linea alba*, and provides the chief point of insertion for the muscles of the lateral abdominal wall.

Make a longitudinal incision in the abdominal wall and attempt to separate the three layers. The external oblique and the internal oblique are fairly well developed and you should be able to distinguish them without difficulty. The transversus is quite thin and may be difficult to separate from the internal oblique.

ORIGINS, INSERTIONS, AND ACTIONS OF THE MUSCLES

(The numbers in parentheses indicate the pages on which the muscles are illustrated.)

Adductor (15). Origin: The ventral surface of the pubis and ischium. Insertion: The distal end of the femur on the medial side. Action: To adduct the hindlimb and to extend the hip.

Anterior deep pectoral (11 and 14). Origin: The anterior portion of the sternum. Insertion: The aponeurosis which covers the supraspinatus at its dorsal end. Action: To adduct and retract the forelimb.

Biceps brachii (14). Origin: The ventral part of the scapula, just above the glenoid fossa. Insertion: The proximal end of the radius and ulna. Action: To flex the e!bow.

Biceps femoris (11). Origin: The lateral portion of the sacrum and ischium. Insertion: By a wide aponeurosis to the patella and the fascia of the thigh and leg. Action: To extend and abduct the hindlimb.

Brachialis (11 and 14). Origin: The proximal third of the humerus. Insertion: The proximal ends of the radius and ulna. Action: To flex the elbow.

Brachiocephalicus (11). Origin: The mastoid process and the nuchal crest. Insertion: The proximal end of the humerus and the fascia of the shoulder. Action: Inclination or extension of the head and neck.

Coracobrachialis (14). Origin: The ventral part of the scapula, just above the glenoid fossa. Insertion: The middle third of the humerus. Action: To adduct the forelimb and flex the shoulder.

Deltoideus (11). Origin: The aponeurosis covering the infraspinatus. Insertion: The proximal end of the humerus and the fascia of the forelimb. Action: To flex the shoulder and abduct the limb.

Digital extensors (forelimb) (11). Origin: The lateral side of the elbow. Insertion: Digits 2–5. Action: To extend the digits and the wrist and to flex the elbow. (This group includes the *common digital extensor, extensor of the second digit,* and *lateral digital extensor.*)

Digital extensors (hindlimb) (11 and 13). Origin: The proximal ends of the fibula and tibia on the lateral side. Insertion: Digits 2–5. Action: To extend the digits and to flex the ankle. (This group includes the *long digital extensor, lateral digital extensor, extensor hallucis longus* and *extensor digitalis brevis.*)

Digital flexors (forelimb) (14). Origin: The distal end of the humerus and the proximal ends of the radius and ulna. Insertion: Digits 2–5. Action: To flex the digits and wrist and to extend the elbow. (This group includes the *superficial digital flexor, deep digital flexor,* and the *flexors of the second and fifth digits.*)

Digital flexors (hindlimb) (11 and 13). Origin: The proximal ends of the fibula and tibia. Insertion: Digits 2–5 . Action: To flex the digits and extend the ankle. (This group includes the *deep* and *superficial digital flexors.*)

Extensor carpi obliquus (11). Origin: The distal two-thirds of the radius and ulna on the lateral side. Insertion: Second metacarpal bone. Action: To extend the wrist.

Extensor carpi radialis (11 and 14). Origin: The distal end of the humerus on the lateral side. Insertion: The third metacarpal bone. Action: To extend and fix the wrist and to flex the elbow.

External oblique (11 and 15). Origin: The lateral surfaces of the ribs behind the fourth, and the lumbodorsal fascia. Insertion: The linea alba, anterior portion of the ilium, and femoral fascia. Action: To compress the abdominal viscera, as in defecation and expiration, and to flex the trunk.

Flexor carpi radialis (14). Origin: The distal end of the humerus on the medial side. Insertion: The third metacarpal bone. Action: To flex the wrist and extend the elbow.

Flexor carpi ulnaris (14). Origin: The distal end of the humerus on the medial side. Insertion: The lateral side of the carpus. Action: To flex the wrist and extend the elbow.

Gastrocnemius and *soleus* (11, 13, and 15). Origin: The distal end of the femur (gastrocnemius) and the head of the fibula (soleus). Insertion: The calcaneus. Action: To extend the ankle or to flex the knee.

Gluteus medius (11 and 13). Origin: The aponeurosis of the longissimus dorsi and the lateral portion of the pelvis. Insertion: The greater trochanter of the femur. Action: To extend the hip and abduct the limb.

Gracilis (15). Origin: The ventral surface of the pubis. Insertion: The proximal third of the tibia on the medial side. Action: To adduct the hindlimb.

Iliacus (13). Origin: The ventral surface of the ilium and the wing of the sacrum. Insertion: The lesser trochanter of the femur, together with the psoas major. Action: To flex the hip and rotate the thigh outward.

Infraspinatus (12). Origin: The lateral side of the scapula posterior to the spine. Insertion: The proximal end of the humerus on the lateral side. Action: To abduct the limb and rotate it outward.

Latissimus dorsi (11). Origin: The four ribs preceding the last. Insertion: The proximal end of the humerus on the medial side. Action: To draw the humerus upward and backward and to flex the shoulder.

Longissimus dorsi (12). Origin: The sacrum, the ilium, and the spinous processes of the lumbar and thoracic vertebrae. Insertion: The transverse processes of the lumbar and thoracic vertebrae, the spinous and transverse processes of the last four cervical vertebrae, and the lateral surfaces of the ribs, except the first. Action: Extension of the back and neck or lateral flexion of the back. The costal attachments may assist in expiration.

Masseter (11). Origin: The zygomatic arch. Insertion: The lateral surface of the mandible. Action: To bring the jaws together.

Pectineus (15). Origin: The anterior border of the pubis. Insertion: The medial side of the femur, about the middle. Action: To adduct the hindlimb and flex the hip.

Psoas major (15). Origin: The ventral sides of the transverse processes of the lumbar vertebrae and the last two ribs. Insertion: The lesser trochanter of the femur, in common with the iliacus. Action: To flex the hip and rotate the thigh outward.

Peroneus longus (11 and 13). Origin: The proximal end of the tibia on the lateral side. Insertion: The first tarsal bone. Action: To flex the ankle.

Peroneus tertius (13 and 15). Origin: The distal end of the femur on the lateral side. Insertion: The third metatarsal and tarsal bones. Action: Mechanically to flex the ankle when the knee is flexed.

Posterior deep pectoral (14). Origin: The ventral side of the sternum and the cartilages of ribs 4–9. Insertion: The proximal end of the humerus. Action: To adduct and retract the limb.

Rectus abdominis (15). Origin: Costal cartilages five through nine, and the adjacent surface of the sternum. Insertion: The pubis. Action: To compress the abdominal viscera, as in defecation and expiration, and to flex the trunk.

Rectus femoris (13 and 15). Origin: The anterior side of the ilium, above the acetabulum. Insertion: The patella. Action: To extend the knee and flex the hip. (Central head of quadriceps femoris.)

Rhomboideus, cephalic part (12). Origin: The occipital bone. Insertion: The dorsal border of the scapula. Action: To draw the scapula forward.

Rhomboideus, cervical, and thoracic parts (12). Origin: The second cervical to the ninth or tenth thoracic vertebrae. Insertion: The dorsal border of the scapula. Action: To draw the scapula upward and forward.

Sartorius (15). Origin: The iliac fascia and the tendon of the psoas minor. Insertion: The proximal end of the tibia on the medial side. Action: To flex the hip and adduct the limb.

Semimembranosus (15). Origin: The ischiac tuberosity. Insertion: The proximal end of the tibia and the distal end of the femur on the medial side. Action: To extend the hip and adduct the hindlimb.

Semitendionsus (13 and 15). Origin: The first and second caudal vertebrae and the ischiac tuberosity. Insertion: The proximal end of the tibia on the medial side, the fascia of the leg, and the calcaneus. Action: To extend the hip.

Serratus ventralis (12). Origin: The cervical vertebrae and the lateral surfaces of the first eight or nine ribs. Insertion: The medial surface of the scapula. Action: To suspend and raise the thorax.

Splenius (12). Origin: Thoracic spines 3, 4, and 5. Insertion: The occipital and temporal bones. Action: To elevate or incline the head and neck.

Sternocephalicus (11, 12, and 14). Origin: The anterior end of the sternum. Insertion: The mastoid process. Action: To flex or incline the head and neck.

Sternothyrohyoideus (11, 12, and 14). Origin: The sternum. Insertion: The laryngeal prominence and the hyoid bone. Action: To retract and depress the hyoid bone, the base of the tongue, and the larynx, as in swallowing.

Superficial pectoral (14). Origin: The ventral side of the sternum. Insertion: The humerus and the fascia of the forelimb. Action: To adduct the forelimb.

Supraspinatus (11 and 12). Origin: The anterior portion of the scapula and the spine of the scapula. Insertion: The proximal end of the humerus on the lateral and anterior sides. Action: To extend the shoulder.

Tensor fasciae latae (11). Origin: The crest of the ilium. Insertion: The *fascia lata*, which is attached to the patella, its ligaments, and the tibia, and is continuous with the fascia covering the superficial muscles on the medial surface of the thigh. Action: To tense the fascia lata, flex the hip, and extend the knee. (The fascia lata is the thick fascia covering the anterior and lateral surfaces of the thigh.)

Teres major (12 and 14). Origin: The posterior border and angle of the scapula. Insertion: The proximal end of the humerus on the medial side, in common with the latissimus dorsi. Action: To flex the shoulder and adduct the limb.

Teres minor (12). Origin: The posterior border of the scapula. Insertion: The proximal end of the humerus on the lateral side. Action: To flex the shoulder, abduct the forelimb, and assist in outward rotation.

Tibialis anterior (13 and 15). Origin: The proximal end of the tibia on the lateral side. Insertion: The second tarsal and metatarsal bones. Action: To flex the ankle.

Trapezius (11). Origin: From the occipital bone to the tenth thoracic vertebra. Insertion: The scapular spine. Action: To elevate the shoulder.

Triceps (11, 12, and 14). Origin: The medial head arises from the proximal third of the humerus on the medial side. The lateral head arises from the proximal end of the humerus on the lateral side. The long head arises from the posterior border of the scapula. Insertion: The three heads insert on the olecranon. Action: To extend the elbow.

Ulnaris lateralis (11). Origin: The distal end of the humerus on the lateral side. Insertion: The fifth metacarpal bone. Action: To flex the wrist and extend the elbow.

Vastus lateralis (13). Origin: The lateral side of the femur. Insertion: The patella and the tendon of the rectus femoris. Action: To extend the knee. (Lateral head of quadriceps femoris.)

Vastus medialis (15). Origin: The proximal two-thirds of the femur on the medial side. Insertion: The patella and the tendon of the rectus femoris. Action: To extend the knee. (Medial head of the quadriceps femoris.)

(The above descriptions of the muscles are based on Sisson's *The Anatomy of Domestic Animals*.)

GLANDS OF THE NECK AND THROAT

Using scissors and being careful to cut only through the skin, make a small V-shaped incision on the lateral side of the head midway between the ear and the mouth. Grasp the point of the V with forceps and pull the skin up, using a scalpel to separate the skin from the underlying structures. Continuing in this manner, skin the lateral side of the head. This must be done very carefully in order not to damage the delicate subcutaneous vessels, glands, and ducts.

Using a binocular loupe or dissecting microscope, dissect away the subcutaneous connective tissue and fat from the structures illustrated on the opposite page. The *duct of the parotid gland*, the *facial nerve*, and the *internal maxillary vein* are surrounded by connective tissue and therefore may be difficult to distinguish, particularly if the veins are not injected. The parotid gland consists of irregular bits of glandular tissue embedded in the subcutaneous connective tissue of the neck and is often difficult to identify because of its immature condition.

Remove the parotid gland and its duct to expose the underlying structures. Beneath the parotid gland are several small *subparotid lymph glands* which should not be confused with the salivary glands. The *duct of the mandibular gland* passes deep through the muscles forming the floor of the mouth and opens near the base of the tongue.

Several ducts from the posterior part of the *sublingual gland* lie near the duct of the mandibular gland but they are small and difficult to identify in the fetal pig. The anterior part of the sublingual gland is much larger than the posterior part. It lies along the base of the tongue beneath the mucous membrane and opens into the floor of the mouth by eight or ten small ducts.

The chief function of the salivary glands is to keep the mouth and pharynx moist. The prominent salivary glands of mammals are associated with the habit of chewing the food, and in man and many other mammals there is an enzyme in the saliva which initiates starch digestion. In birds, reptiles, and amphibians, most of which take their food with little chewing, the salivary glands are not as well developed as they are in mammals.

In frogs, the mucous membrane of the tongue contains numerous mucus-secreting glands, and an *intermaxillary gland* in the anterior part of the mouth produces the sticky secretion which makes insects adhere to the frog's tongue.

Refer to page 24 and identify the *thymus gland*. It is prominent in young animals, but atrophies after puberty and is usually not distinguishable in mature animals. The thymus is a primary center for the production of *lymphocytes*, the most abundant of the wandering cells. Lymphocytes are liberated from the thymus into the bloodstream and settle in such organs as the spleen and lymph nodes. Experimental evidence indicates that, within the thymus, lymphocytes are differentiated into groups with varying immunological potentials, and that the descendants of the lymphocytes liberated from the thymus produce antibodies responsible for the body's ability to resist infection and disease.

Identify the *thyroid gland*. It is an oval body lying in the midline and covered by the cervical part of the thymus gland. The thyroid gland produces *thyroxin*, a hormone which affects metabolic rate, growth, and differentiation, as well as exercising an influence upon other endocrine glands. Disturbances of thyroid function in humans result in metabolic irregularity and disorders such as cretinism (associated with deficient thyroid hormone production) and exophthalmic goiter (associated with excessive production of the thyroid hormone). Temperature is the chief environmental factor influencing thyroid activity. This, together with the fact that administration of thyroxin increases metabolism in terrestrial vertebrates (but not in fish), suggests that the thyroid gland played an important role in the evolution of intrinsic temperature control.

The thymus and thyroid glands are both present in frogs. The role of the thymus in the frog has been little studied, but the effects of the thyroid hormone on the metamorphosis of tadpoles has been the subject of considerable research. Tadpoles fed with thyroid extract metamorphose quickly into small frogs, but tadpoles in which the thyroid gland has been removed do not metamorphose at all.

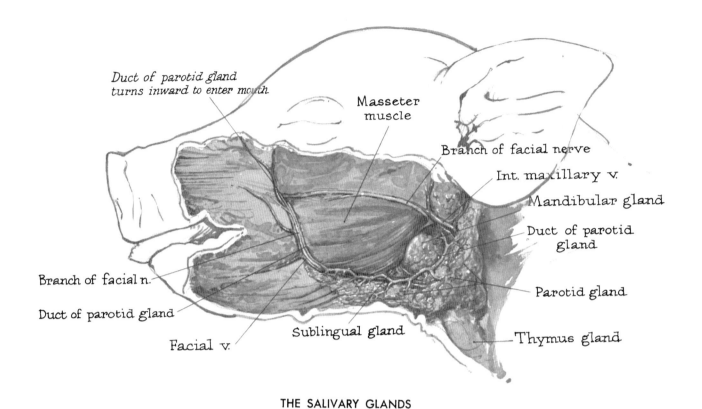

Duct of parotid gland
turns inward to enter mouth

Masseter
muscle

Branch of facial nerve

Int. maxillary v.

Mandibular gland

Duct of parotid
gland

Parotid gland

Thymus gland

Branch of facial n.

Duct of parotid gland

Facial v.

Sublingual gland

THE SALIVARY GLANDS

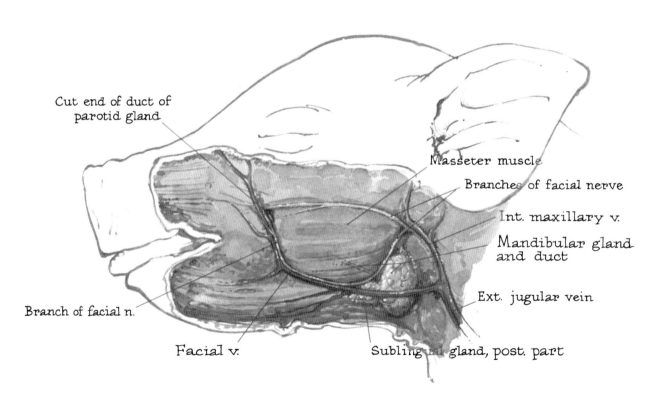

Cut end of duct of
parotid gland

Masseter muscle

Branches of facial nerve

Int. maxillary v.

Mandibular gland
and duct

Ext. jugular vein

Branch of facial n.

Facial v.

Sublingual gland, post. part

The parotid gland and its duct are removed to show
underlying structures.

THE ORAL CAVITY

Use bone clippers and a knife to cut the angles of the jaw and expose the oral cavity. Identify the structures illustrated on the opposite page. Trim away the soft palate to find the internal nares and the openings of the Eustachian tubes.

Because of their immature condition, identification of the teeth in the fetal pig will be difficult and they may best be identified in the cat skull.

Notice that the mouth of the frog is relatively larger in relation to the head and body than the mouth of the pig. The frog uses its tongue to snare insects and flip them back into its mouth, and so the bigger the mouth, the easier it is to get food into it. Large mouths have evolved independently in such unrelated insect-eaters as the frog, swift, and bat.

In comparing the tongues of the frog and the pig, observe that whereas the tongue of the frog is attached at the front of the mouth, the tongue of the pig, like that of most other vertebrates, is attached at the back of the mouth. The anterior attachment of the frog's tongue is part of the remarkable tongue-flipping mechanism which enables it to catch an insect on the wing.

A frog cannot drink through a straw; it lacks the *secondary palate* and the mobile lips and cheeks associated with the sucking and chewing habits of mammals. When a young mammal nurses, the suction within the mouth draws the base of the tongue against the *soft palate*, forming an airtight partition between the mouth and *pharynx* so that while milk is drawn into the front of the mouth, air passes freely through the nose and into the lungs. When the mouth is full of milk the tongue relaxes, opening the partition between the oral cavity and the pharynx. The *epiglottis* folds back over the *glottis*, closing off the entrance to the *trachea*, breathing is interrupted for a moment, and milk passes from the mouth into the *esophagus*. When the mammal is old enough to take solid food, the hard and soft palates provide a partition between the mouth and nasal passages, making it possible for the animal to breathe while there is food in the mouth.

The high metabolic rate of mammals makes constant breathing a necessity. It would be almost impossible for a mammal to stop breathing while it chewed its food. Frogs, because of their low metabolic rate, can survive for long periods without using their lungs, and they experience no difficulty in suspending pulmonary respiration for the short time it takes to flip a worm or insect into the mouth. In frogs, therefore, a secondary palate is unnecessary. The nares open directly into the anterior part of the oral cavity and there is neither hard palate, soft palate, nor epiglottis.

The secondary palate of mammals also serves to keep food and drink away from the olfactory area, which is more highly developed in mammals than in amphibians and reptiles. The frog, which depends chiefly on vision for locating its prey, has a relatively small olfactory area. The size of the *nasal conchae* and the presence of a secondary palate are skeletal features which paleontologists use as a basis for estimating the degree of warm-bloodedness attained by certain fossil forms.

The teeth of mammals are far fewer and more specialized than the numerous small conical teeth typical of fish, reptiles, and amphibians. The reduction in the number of the teeth with the evolution of mammals is an example of an evolutionary process known as *Williston's law:* "The parts of an organism tend toward reduction in number, with the fewer parts greatly specialized in function." Examples of this process may be found in many evolutionary sequences. Primitive crustaceans such as the trilobites had many similar segments and legs, whereas modern crustaceans such as lobsters and crabs have legs which are far fewer and more specialized. In fishes the basic plan is to use a few elements over and over. The W-shaped muscle segments, the vertebrae, and the fin rays are repeated with only minor variations. In mammals, structural features are for the most part fewer and more specialized. The many similar rays of the fish's pectoral and pelvic fins are represented in mammals by the highly specialized bones of the legs. The vertebrae, ribs, skull bones, and teeth of mammals are in most cases fewer and more highly specialized than those of primitive vertebrates, and except for the intercostal muscles (homologs of the ventral trunk muscles of fishes), each bilaterally symmetrical pair of muscles in the mammal is unique.

Because of its small teeth, the frog cannot attack animals of any size, nor can it eat vegetable food, which requires grinding and chewing. The omnivorous pig, in contrast, is a fierce fighter equipped with formidable cutting teeth and also with molars for grinding vegetable food. These adaptations enable the pig to eat a far greater variety of food than the frog can eat; perhaps the one form of food the pig cannot effectively pursue is an insect on the wing.

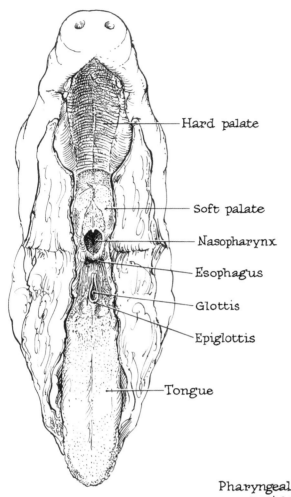

Hard palate

Soft palate

Nasopharynx

Esophagus

Glottis

Epiglottis

Tongue

The jaws are cut to reveal the oral cavity.

	Incisors	Canines	Premolars	Molars		Incisors	Canines	Premolars	Molars	
	3	1	3	1		3	1	4	3	Upper jaw
	3	1	2	1		3	1	4	3	Lower jaw
		Cat					Pig			

THE DENTAL FORMULA

This formula is used as a shorthand device for comparing the teeth of various mammals. Note that the premolars and molars, specialized for chewing vegetable food, are more numerous in the omnivorous pig than in the carnivorous cat.

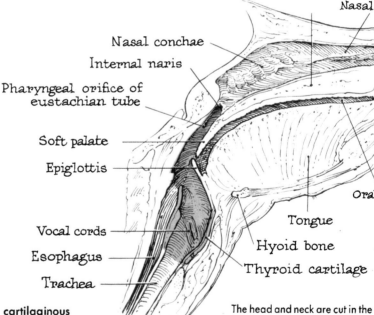

Hard palate

Nasal cavity

Nasal conchae

Internal naris

Pharyngeal orifice of eustachian tube

Soft palate

Epiglottis

Vocal cords

Esophagus

Trachea

Oral cavity

Tongue

Hyoid bone

Thyroid cartilage

The head and neck are cut in the sagittal plane and the nasal septum is removed.

The larynx (blue), or organ of voice, is a cartilaginous structure containing the vocal cords. The epiglottis is a flexible cartilage which covers the glottis (the opening between the trachea and the pharynx) when food is swallowed. The pharynx (red) is a saclike portion of the digestive tube at the cranial end of the esophagus. The internal nares, Eustachian tubes, mouth, larynx, and esophagus open into it. The pharynx is divided into two parts: the nasopharynx, dorsal to the soft palate, and the oropharynx, between the soft palate and the level of the hyoid bone.

21

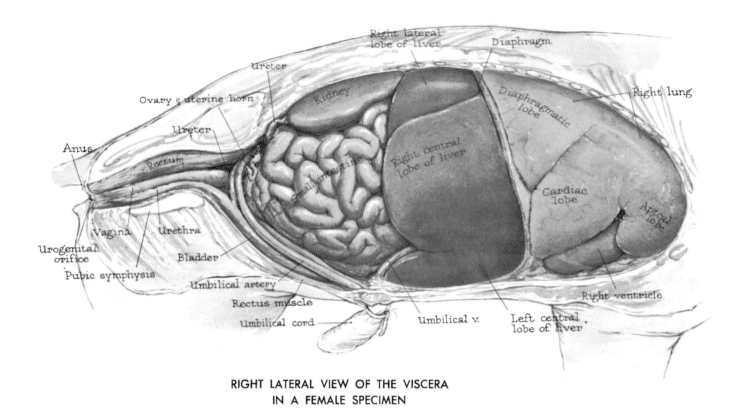

**RIGHT LATERAL VIEW OF THE VISCERA
IN A FEMALE SPECIMEN**

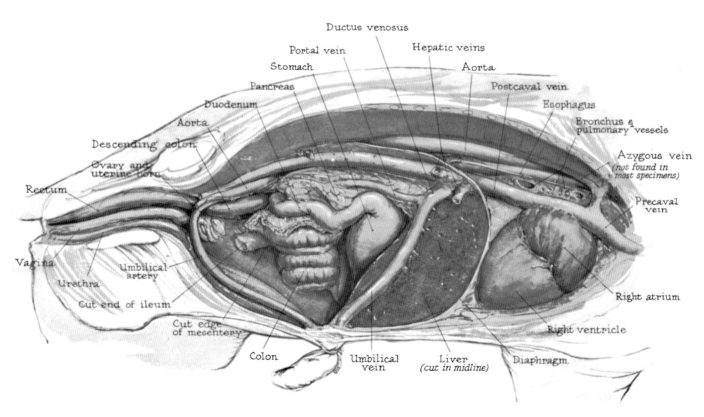

The small intestine, right half of the
liver, and right lung are removed.

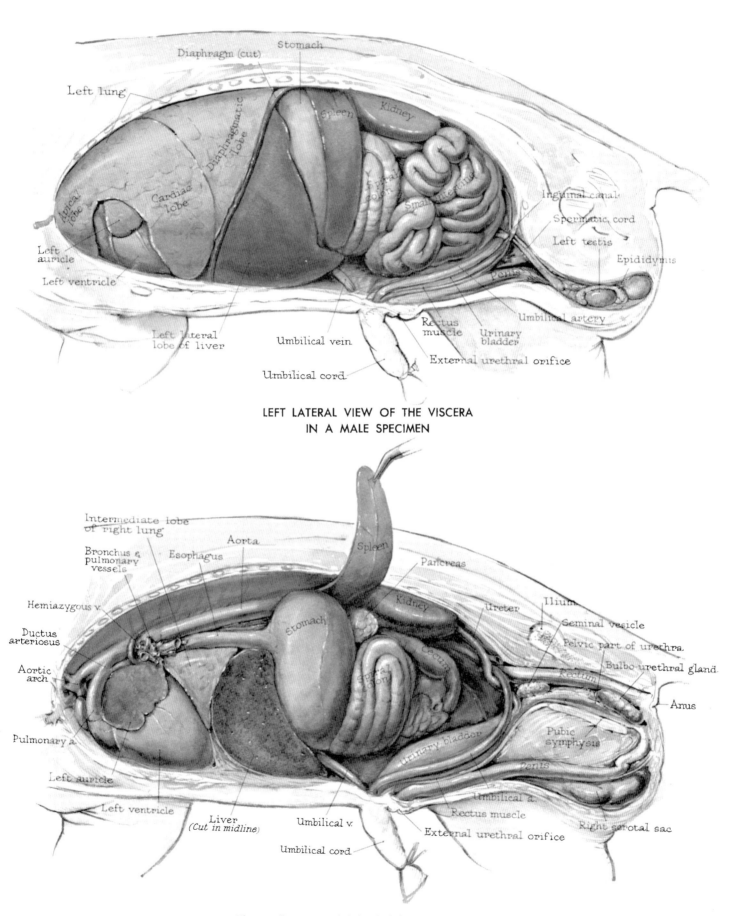

Diaphragm (cut)

Stomach

Left lung

Spleen

Kidney

Diaphragmatic lobe

Apical lobe

Cardiac lobe

Spiral colon

Small intestine

Inguinal canal

Spermatic cord

Left auricle

Left testis

Left ventricle

Epididymus

Penis

Rectus muscle

Umbilical artery

Left lateral lobe of liver

Umbilical vein

Urinary bladder

Umbilical cord

External urethral orifice

LEFT LATERAL VIEW OF THE VISCERA
IN A MALE SPECIMEN

Intermediate lobe of right lung

Aorta

Bronchus & pulmonary vessels

Esophagus

Spleen

Pancreas

Hemiazygous v.

Kidney

Ureter

Ilium

Ductus arteriosus

Stomach

Seminal vesicle

Pelvic part of urethra

Aortic arch

Cecum

Bulbo-urethral gland

Spiral colon

Rectum

Anus

Pulmonary a.

Urinary bladder

Pubic symphysis

Left auricle

Penis

Left ventricle

Liver (Cut in midline)

Umbilical v.

Umbilical a.

Rectus muscle

Right scrotal sac

External urethral orifice

Umbilical cord

The small intestine, left half of the
liver, and left lung are removed

23

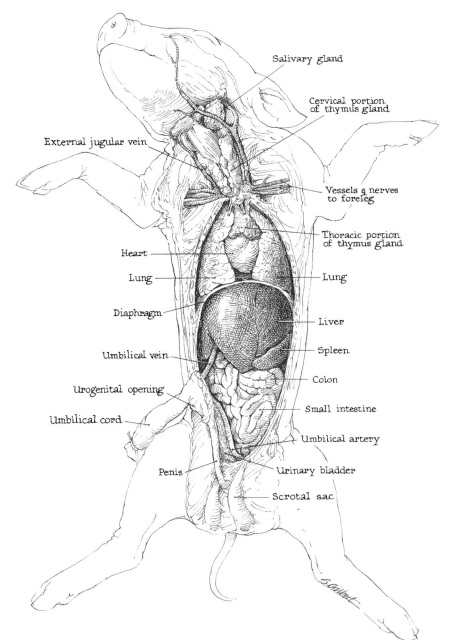

Salivary gland

Cervical portion of thymus gland

External jugular vein

Vessels & nerves to foreleg

Thoracic portion of thymus gland

Heart

Lung

Lung

Diaphragm

Liver

Spleen

Umbilical vein

Colon

Urogenital opening

Small intestine

Umbilical cord

Umbilical artery

Penis

Urinary bladder

Scrotal sac

THE DIGESTIVE SYSTEM

Tie your specimen to the dissecting pan as directed for the ventral dissection of the muscles. If no dissection of the muscles was made, and if your specimen is a male, remove the skin in the midline posterior to the umbilical cord and identify the penis and the scrotal sacs before you open the body cavity. Refer to the illustrations on pages 23 and 33 as you do this.

In opening the *abdominal* and *thoracic cavities*, be sure you are cutting only through the body wall and not injuring any of the underlying structures. Cut slowly, lifting up the edge of the cut as you go and watching the points of the scissors. You will find it helpful to refer to the lateral views on pages 22 and 23 to see the underlying structures as you follow the instructions for opening the abdomen and the thorax.

Insert one point of your scissors in the midline just anterior to the umbilical cord and cut through the rectus muscle. Continue your cut toward the head, using stout scissors to cut through the sternum. Do not extend the cut farther than the anterior end of the sternum. Now start at the umbilical cord, cut around it, and continue this cut to the pelvis, keeping somewhat to the side of the midline to avoid the bladder.

Cut the umbilical vein near the lower margin of the liver. Starting at the anterior end of the rib cage and working toward the pelvis on either side, trim away the thoracic and abdominal walls to expose the viscera. Leave the umbilical cord, bladder, umbilical arteries, and penis intact. Wash out any latex or organic debris which may be found in the abdominal cavity. Your dissection should now look like the above illustration.

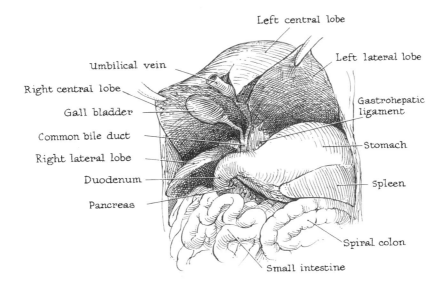

Left central lobe

Left lateral lobe

Umbilical vein

Right central lobe

Gall bladder

Gastrohepatic ligament

Common bile duct

Stomach

Right lateral lobe

Duodenum

Spleen

Pancreas

Spiral colon

Small intestine

Before doing any further dissecting, explore the relations of the abdominal viscera by gently pushing them first to one side and then to the other, and by lifting the *liver* and the *stomach*. As you do this refer to the lateral views and to the other illustrations in this section. Identify the organs and form an understanding of their general relations, but do not concern yourself with the identification of ducts, ligaments, or vessels at this time.

Explore the extent of the *diaphragm* and observe that it consists of a central *tendinous portion* from which muscular fibers extend to the body wall. During inspiration, the ribs are raised and the diaphragm contracts, forcing the abdominal viscera downward. In this way, the size of the thoracic cavity is increased in two directions at once.

Because of its low metabolic rate, the frog breathes infrequently and can survive by occasionally pumping air into the lungs with its mouth. In frogs, we find neither the movable ribs nor the diaphragm which are associated with the constant and rapid breathing of mammals.

Observe the thin, semiopaque membrane on the abdominal surface of the diaphragm. This is the *peritoneum*, which lines the entire abdominal cavity and its contents, as well as forming the *mesenteries* and *ligaments* between the viscera and the abdominal wall. The portion of the peritoneum which covers the viscera is called the *visceral peritoneum*, whereas the portion lining the abdominal wall is called the *parietal peritoneum*. The potential space between the visceral and parietal peritoneum is the abdominal or *peritoneal cavity*; this cavity is a subdivision of the *celom*, or body cavity of the embryo. The celom also gives rise to the cavities containing the heart and lungs.

Raise the *liver* and identify the structures illustrated above. Separate the fibers of the *gastrohepatic ligament* with a dull probe and identify the *common bile duct*. Referring to the illustration of the visceral surface of the liver on page 26, also identify the *cystic duct* and the *hepatic duct*. If the *umbilical vein* in your specimen contains injected latex, look for the *portal vein* just dorsal to the common bile duct. Explore the anterior surface of the liver and find the *postcaval vein* extending between the liver and the heart.

Look at the lateral views of the liver on pages 22 and 47, and study the relations of the umbilical vein, postcaval vein, portal vein, and *ductus venosus*. If the umbilical vein in your specimen is injected, you may attempt to trace these veins by picking away the substance of the liver on the right side to make a dissection resembling that on page 22. If the umbilical vein is not injected, it will not be practical to trace the course of the veins within the liver.

The external form of the liver has no particular significance; it is an organ which adapts itself to the space it fills and its shape may vary considerably. There are, however, four significant structural features which should be observed in dissection:

1. The liver is a very vascular organ, as is demonstrated by the fact that when you cut into its substance you will find it full of latex strands.

2. The bile ducts connect the liver to the alimentary canal.

3. The portal vein passes from the alimentary canal to the liver, where it divides into many branches.

4. The hepatic veins enter the postcaval vein within the

liver. In the adult, blood from the portal vein passes through the capillaries and sinuses of the liver before returning to the postcaval vein via the hepatic veins. The ductus venosus and the umbilical vein are fetal structures which close after birth.

The liver is the first stop and main storage depot for nutriment carried by the blood from the intestine. The liver has many functions, including the storage, modification, and release of glycogen and other blood constituents. It also transforms waste products of protein metabolism into nontoxic compounds which are returned to the blood to be excreted by the kidneys. Other products of protein decomposition pass from the liver into the alimentary canal as *bile*, which is stored in the *gall bladder* and conveyed by the bile ducts. Bile contains no digestive enzymes but it does contain certain salts which are functional in the breakdown and absorption of fats.

The functions of the liver are similar in the pig and the frog. Of course, in the frog there is neither umbilical vein nor ductus venosus; the tadpole develops outside the maternal body, carrying on respiratory exchange directly with the environment and receiving nutriment from the yolk of the egg. Perhaps the most striking difference between the livers of the frog and the pig is that the liver of the pig remains constant in size throughout the year whereas the frog's liver reaches a maximum size in early fall and grows gradually smaller during the winter until by spring it is only about one-half to one-third of its former size. In the frog, nutriment is stored in the fat bodies and in the liver, both of which decrease markedly in size as their food stores are depleted during hibernation. Because frogs are cold-blooded, they store nutriment inside the body cavity instead of storing it as subcutaneous fat. The subcutaneous layer of fat which serves as heat-retaining insulation for the mammal would be of no use to the frog. Subcutaneous fat in a frog would interfere with cutaneous respiration, cutaneous water absorption, and, most important, would act as insulation against the absorption of heat from the environment.

Remove the liver by cutting the postcaval vein, the portal vein, the common bile duct, and the connective tissue and peritoneal attachments which hold it to the body wall. If you did not destroy half of the liver by tracing the course of the umbilical and portal veins, remove it intact. Study the visceral surface and identify the structures illustrated above.

Lift the stomach and clear away the thin peritoneal membrane beneath it to find the *pancreas* (see page 29). The pancreas produces enzymes which function in the digestion of fats, proteins, and carbohydrates. These enzymes enter the alimentary canal via the *pancreatic duct*, which opens into the duodenum just distal to the opening of the com-

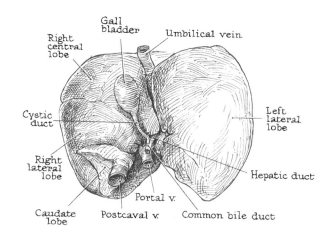

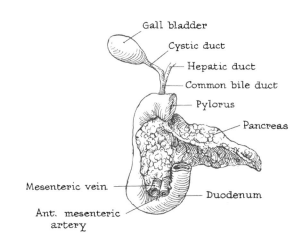

mon bile duct. Other digestive enzymes are produced in the small intestine. The pancreas also produces a hormone, *insulin*, which is secreted directly into the blood. Insulin plays a vital role in the regulation of carbohydrate metabolism. Low insulin production results in diabetes, a condition in which liver storage of glycogen decreases and sugar is eliminated unused by the kidneys.

The *spleen* is a lymphatic organ. In adult mammals, erythrocytes are stored and destroyed in the spleen, and lymphocytes are formed in it. In the fetal spleen both erythrocytes and leukocytes are formed, and this function persists in adult amphibians and reptiles. Other functions of the mammalian spleen are not fully understood. It may be removed without fatal results, which is not true of the pancreas or the liver.

Pull the *small intestine* to the right and examine the *mesentery* which attaches it to the dorsal body wall. Within the mesentery, observe the rich blood supply and the many *lymph glands* which appear as small white lobulated structures near the point at which the mesentery is attached to the dorsal body wall. These lymph glands are associated with the *mesenteric lymphatics* or *lacteals*. Lymph almost always passes through at least one set of lymph glands before returning to the bloodstream. The mesenteric veins and lymphatics are the routes by which absorbed nutriment begins its passage from the intestine to its various destinations. Carbohydrates and proteins pass into the intestinal capillaries and then via the mesenteric and portal veins to the liver and other parts of the body, but most fats enter the circulation by way of the lymphatics. It is thought that this is because the lymphatics are more permeable to the relatively large fat molecules than are capillaries.

Now cut the distal end of the *duodenum* near the *duodenojejunal junction* as illustrated on page 28 (cut 1). Cut the mesentery of the small intestine near its origin, cut the *ileum* near the *ileocecal junction* (cut 2), and remove the small intestine. Your dissection should now resemble the illustration on page 28.

Now refer to page 29. Cut the *esophagus* just above the *stomach* (cut 3) and cut the proximal end of the duodenum just distal to the pylorus (cut 4). Remove the stomach and spleen. Press the *spiral part of the colon* to the right and cut the colon at the point where the spiral part merges with the *ascending part* (cut 5). Dissect away the peritoneum which covers the remaining parts of the duodenum and colon so that your dissection resembles the illustration on page 29.

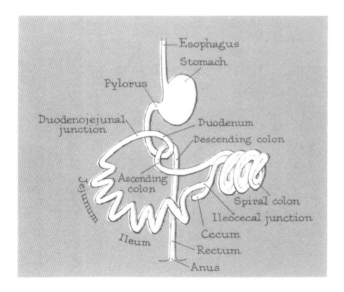

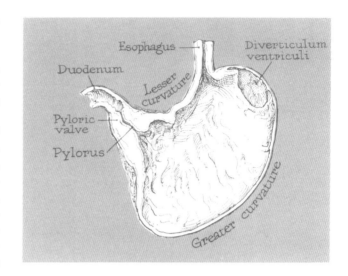

Cut open the stomach along the *greater* and *lesser curvatures* and identify the parts illustrated above.

Cut open a section of the *jejunum*, place it in a shallow dish of water, and examine it under a lens or dissecting microscope. The velvety appearance of the mucosa in the small intestine is due to the presence of minute projections termed *villi*, which increase the absorptive area of the intestinal mucosa much as the texture of a turkish towel increases the absorptive area of cloth. Cut open and examine a section of the *descending colon*. Notice that villi are present in the small intestine, but not in the stomach or colon. This is because the absorption of nutriment occurs only in the small intestine.

Notice that the alimentary canal is relatively longer in the pig than it is in the frog and that villi are not found in the intestine of the frog. The presence of villi in the pig's intestine provides up to fifteen times more absorptive surface than a comparable section of frog intestine. The villi represent an adaptation related to the high metabolic rate and large food intake of mammals. Another factor affecting the relatively large intestinal area of the pig is the fact that the pig is omnivorous. The intestinal tracts of herbivorous and omnivorous animals are characteristically longer than those of meat eaters, which get their food in more concentrated form and therefore do not need such an extensive intestinal area. The alimentary canal of the omnivorous tadpole just before metamorphosis is over twice as long as that of the young carnivorous frog just after metamorphosis.

It is sometimes said that small animals have relatively short alimentary canals, whereas large animals have relatively long ones. This difference is explained by reference to surface-volume relationships by using some such analogy as this: In a rotifer, a straight intestine is adequate to absorb the required nutriment because the surface of the

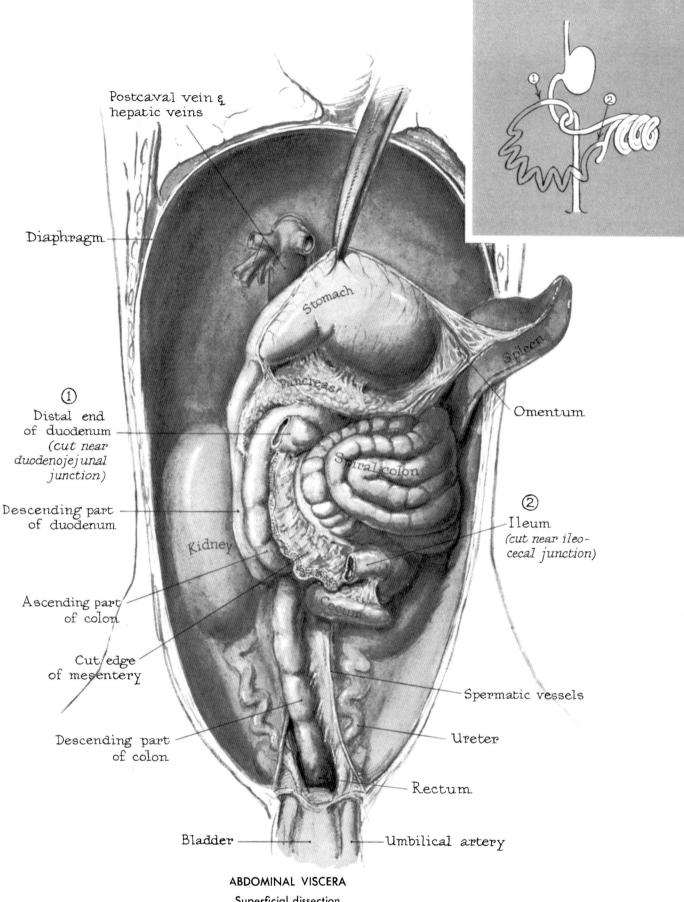

Postcaval vein &
hepatic veins

Diaphragm

Stomach

Pancreas

Spleen

Omentum

① Distal end
of duodenum
(cut near
duodenojejunal
junction)

Descending part
of duodenum

Spiral colon

② Ileum
(cut near ileo-
cecal junction)

Kidney

Ascending part
of colon

Cecum

Cut edge
of mesentery

Spermatic vessels

Descending part
of colon

Ureter

Rectum

Bladder

Umbilical artery

ABDOMINAL VISCERA
Superficial dissection

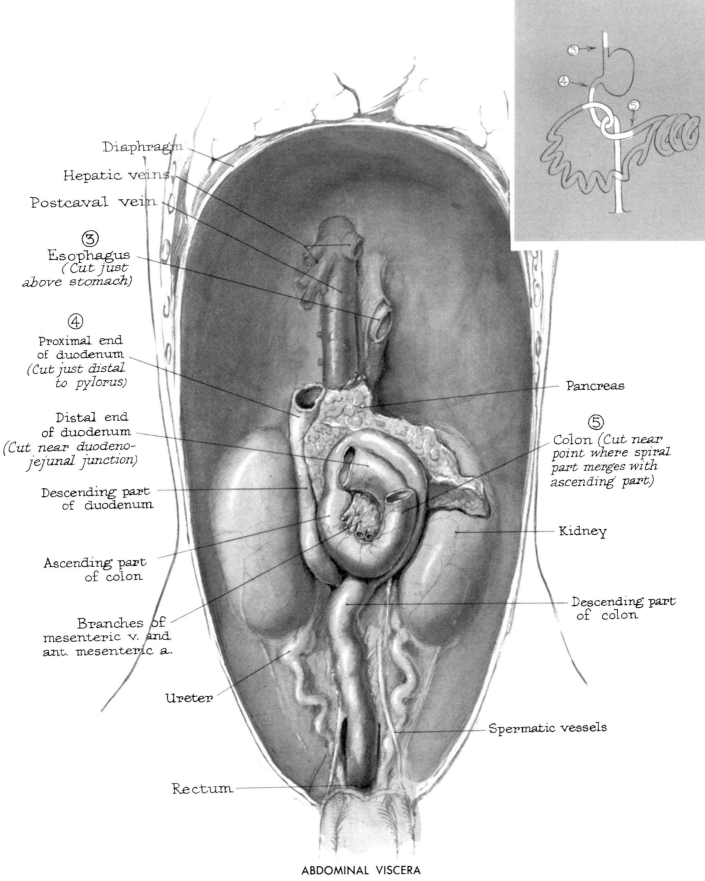

Diaphragm

Hepatic veins

Postcaval vein

③
Esophagus
(Cut just
above stomach)

④
Proximal end
of duodenum
(Cut just distal
to pylorus)

Distal end
of duodenum
(Cut near duodeno-
jejunal junction)

Descending part
of duodenum

Ascending part
of colon

Branches of
mesenteric v. and
ant. mesenteric a.

Ureter

Rectum

Pancreas

⑤
Colon (Cut near
point where spiral
part merges with
ascending part)

Kidney

Descending part
of colon

Spermatic vessels

ABDOMINAL VISCERA
Deep dissection

intestine is relatively large in relation to the volume of the animal. If we were to increase the length of the rotifer by ten times, its volume would increase by a factor of one thousand while the absorptive area of the intestine would increase by a factor of only one hundred. The giant rotifer would either have to absorb ten times more food through each square inch of intestine or else deliver one-tenth as much nutriment to each cubic inch of tissue.

On the basis of this imaginary construction, we would expect to find a disproportionate increase in the respiratory, absorptive, and excretory surfaces of large animals. We might observe that a rotifer can get along with a straight intestine and relatively simple excretory organs, while its body surface provides area enough for the exchange of respiratory gases, whereas man, with his volume increased all out of proportion to his respiratory, absorptive, and excretory surfaces, needs one hundred square yards of lung surface (sixty-six times the body surface), twelve square yards of intestinal mucosa (seven-and-one-half times the body surface), and somewhat under one square yard of glomerular filtering surface in the kidney (about half the body surface). From this we might conclude that the alimentary canal of the pig is disproportionately longer than the alimentary canal of the frog because the volume of the body requiring nutriment is disproportionately greater in the pig.

Actual measurements, however, show that this conclusion is untenable. The absorptive surface of man's intestine is not disproportionately larger than the absorptive surface of a rat's intestine. The man weighs one thousand times as much as the rat but his intestinal surface is only about one hundred times that of the rat. In comparing the intestinal surfaces of the planaria, roundworm, earthworm, frog, and shark we do *not* find the disproportionate increases in the digestive and respiratory surfaces which the analogy of the giant rotifer would lead us to expect. Measurements show that although there are many individual variations, intestinal and respiratory surfaces tend to be more nearly proportional to total body surface than to total body weight. Because of their high metabolic rate and large food intake, warm-blooded animals have longer alimentary canals than cold-blooded animals of comparable size, but large warm-blooded animals do not, in general, have disproportionately longer alimentary canals than small warm-blooded animals, nor do large cold-blooded animals have disproportionately longer alimentary canals than small cold-blooded animals.

As we saw in our discussion of the relation between temperature, volume, and surface, large mammals produce less heat per pound than small ones. In a rat, both the area of the skin and the area of the intestine are large in relation to the volume. The large intake of food produces a great deal of heat, most of which is dissipated through the large skin surface. In man, both the area of the intestine and the body surface are much smaller in relation to the volume. Less heat is lost through the skin and a smaller intake of food is sufficient to maintain approximately the same body temperature.

To put it differently: one thousand rats weigh as much as a man, have a total skin area about ten times that of a man, dissipate about ten times as much heat through the skin as a man does, and replace the dissipated heat by eating ten times as much food, which is absorbed through ten times the intestinal surface.

We know that among cold-blooded animals, too, large individuals have lower metabolic rates than small individuals. We also know that in them the dissipation of internally produced heat through the body surface is negligible and therefore it might be expected that metabolic rates of cold-blooded animals would be proportional to some factor other than body surface. Measurements show that this is the case in very small cold-blooded animals: among unicellular organisms and among some insect larva and adults, metabolism is directly proportional to weight. In many cold-blooded animals, however, metabolism is directly proportional to body surface; in others it is nearly so. When large samples of warm-blooded animals, cold-blooded animals, and plants are plotted over a wide range of sizes it is found that metabolism is more nearly proportional to body surface than to weight; if a small animal consumes x units of oxygen for every unit of surface area, a large animal will consume slightly more than x units of oxygen for every unit of surface area.

Many factors are involved in the approximate correlation between body surface and metabolism. These factors are not fully understood and no simple explanation of this relationship is possible. Numerous explanations have, however, been attempted. One of the most common is to imagine what would happen if metabolism were, in fact, directly proportional to weight. If this were true, the disproportionate proliferation of the surfaces across which metabolic exchange occurs would be so tremendous in large organisms that all large organisms would be radically different in appearance from all small organisms. Of course, this is not the case. A small fish is similar in external and internal form to a large fish; this would not be true if metabolism were not very nearly proportional to body surface.

Another argument is found in the familiar example of heat dissipation through body surface. If metabolism were directly proportional to weight, large organisms would be much warmer than small organisms, and this would be true of cold-blooded animals and plants as well as of warm-blooded animals. Such temperature differences are not found in nature. The body temperature of a ten-ton shark is very nearly the same as that of the smallest teleost (*Schindleria*, 2 mg) when both are swimming in the same water, and this would not be true if metabolism were not very nearly proportional to body surface.

If metabolism were directly proportional to weight, all ecological relations would be radically changed. Food intake, like metabolism, is approximately proportional to body surface. If it were proportional to weight, large animals would require tremendous quantities of nourishment and would be much scarcer than they are.

The functional interdependence of surface, volume, and metabolism is related to many aspects of biological form and function, and is one of the most basic considerations in the comparison of organic forms. An introduction to this fascinating topic may be found in A. M. Hemmingsen's extensive survey: "The Relation of Standard (Basal) Energy Metabolism to Total Fresh Weight of Living Organisms," published in the *Reports of the Steno Memorial Hospital* (1950), 4:7–58.

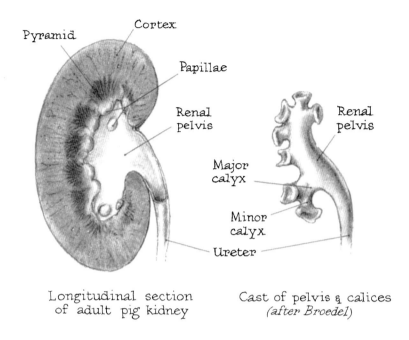

Pyramid

Cortex

Papillae

Renal pelvis

Major calyx

Minor calyx

Ureter

Renal pelvis

Longitudinal section
of adult pig kidney

Cast of pelvis & calices
(after Broedel)

THE KIDNEYS AND ADRENAL GLANDS

Remove the pancreas and the remaining portions of the duodenum and the descending colon, being careful to avoid injury to the underlying vessels. Then remove the peritoneum and connective tissue from the ventral surface of the aorta, postcaval vein, and kidneys. These structures lie on the dorsal body wall and are covered by peritoneum only on the ventral side. They are therefore said to be *retroperitoneal*, or behind the peritoneum, in contrast to structures such as the spleen, jejunum, ileum, and liver, which lie within the central part of the abdominal cavity and are almost completely surrounded by their peritoneal coverings.

If your specimen is a male, refer to the opposite page and identify the structures illustrated. If your specimen is a female, identify the structures illustrated on page 41, but do not cut the pubic symphysis or remove the uterus and vagina until instructed to do so.

Make a longitudinal section of an adult mammalian kidney and identify the structures illustrated above.

The *adrenals* are glands of internal secretion and have no direct physiological connection with the kidneys, although hormones produced in the adrenals do affect kidney function among other things. The adrenal gland consists of two parts, an outer *cortex* and an inner *medulla* (not grossly distinguishable in the fetal pig). These two parts have different embryological origins and different functions.

The cortex produces a number of hormones which influence sexual development and behavior, metabolism, and the water-salt balance of the blood and interstitial fluids. The adrenal medulla produces the well-known hormone *epinephrine*, which effects a number of emergency reactions such as raising the blood pressure and increasing blood sugar and cardiac output. Synthetically prepared epinephrine is sold under a variety of trade names (*adrenalin* among them) and is used as a vasoconstrictor in hemorrhage, to relax pulmonary bronchial muscles in cases of bronchitis or asthma, to prolong the effects of local anesthetics, and in the treatment of shock.

In the frog, the adrenal gland is seen as an irregular, flattened band of tissue adhering closely to the ventral side of the kidney throughout its length, with the homologs of the cortex and medulla mingled instead of separated into inner and outer layers. This represents a transitional stage; in fishes, the homologs of the cortex and medulla are completely separate structures which lie along the length of the dorsal body wall near the kidneys.

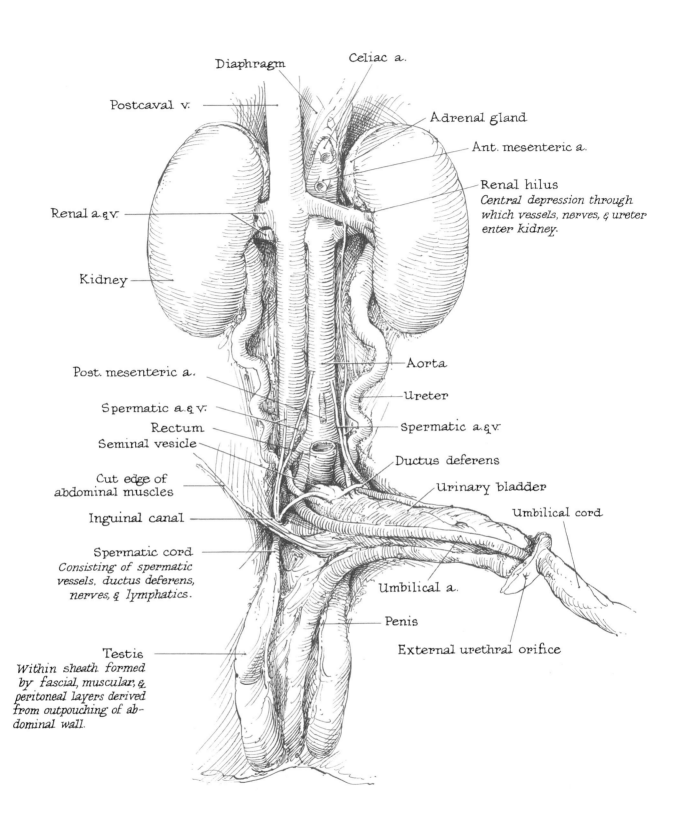

Diaphragm

Celiac a.

Postcaval v.

Adrenal gland

Ant. mesenteric a.

Renal hilus
*Central depression through
which vessels, nerves, & ureter
enter kidney.*

Renal a. & v.

Kidney

Post. mesenteric a.

Aorta

Ureter

Spermatic a. & v.

Rectum

Spermatic a. & v.

Seminal vesicle

Ductus deferens

Cut edge of
abdominal muscles

Urinary bladder

Umbilical cord

Inguinal canal

Spermatic cord
*Consisting of spermatic
vessels, ductus deferens,
nerves, & lymphatics.*

Umbilical a.

Penis

External urethral orifice

Testis
*Within sheath formed
by fascial, muscular, &
peritoneal layers derived
from outpouching of ab-
dominal wall.*

THE MALE UROGENITAL SYSTEM

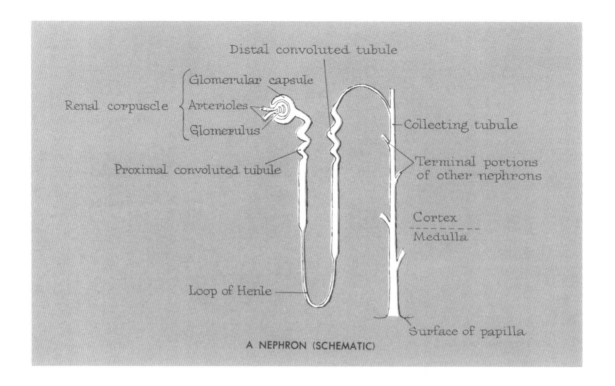

Distal convoluted tubule

Renal corpuscle {
  Glomerular capsule
  Arterioles
  Glomerulus
}

Collecting tubule

Terminal portions of other nephrons

Proximal convoluted tubule

Cortex
——————
Medulla

Loop of Henle

Surface of papilla

A NEPHRON (SCHEMATIC)

THE WORK OF THE KIDNEYS

An environment which is thermally and chemically stable within fairly narrow limits is essential for animal metabolism. The ocean provides such an environment for marine protozoa, which exchange metabolic input and output directly with their external environment. Every living cell in the body of a terrestrial vertebrate is surrounded by an *internal environment* similar in composition to dilute sea water. The cells of a terrestrial vertebrate exchange metabolic input and output with their internal environment just as the unicellular marine organism exchanges with its external environment.

The internal environment is defined as the *extracellular fluid*, or the sum total of all body fluid *outside* the cells; this includes the fluid components of the blood and lymph as well as all body fluids surrounding the cells. The extracellular fluid is the medium through which every cell exchanges oxygen, nutriment, and metabolic wastes with the outside world. As the fluid component of blood, it flows through the arteries and veins carrying blood cells, proteins, and fats. Minus these elements, it filters through the capillary walls, bathes every living cell of the body, and is returned again to the blood-circulatory system via the lymphatics. Any change in the volume or composition

of the extracellular fluid has drastic effects, and its constant regulation by the kidneys is therefore one of the most important operations in the economy of the body.

The functional units of the kidney are minute membranous tubules termed *nephrons*. A single human kidney contains about a million nephrons which follow an intricate course in the cortex and medulla, finally emptying into *collecting tubules* which open onto the *renal papillae*. All the blood from the *renal artery* goes through the capillaries of the nephrons before returning to the *renal vein*.

When blood enters the *glomerulus* (the capillary unit of the *renal corpuscle*) the blood cells, proteins, and fats remain in the capillaries but the extracellular fluid, together with its solutes, filters into the *glomerular capsule*. As this fluid passes through the nephron, most of it is reabsorbed into the bloodstream by the *peritubular capillaries*. This process is termed *tubular reabsorption*. The metabolic wastes and excess water which are not reabsorbed pass into the collecting tubules and from there to the *renal pelvis*, *ureter*, and *urinary bladder*.

The processes of glomerular filtration and tubular reabsorption are supplemented by *tubular excretion*, which is the transfer of certain substances from the blood in the peritubular capillaries directly into the nephron.

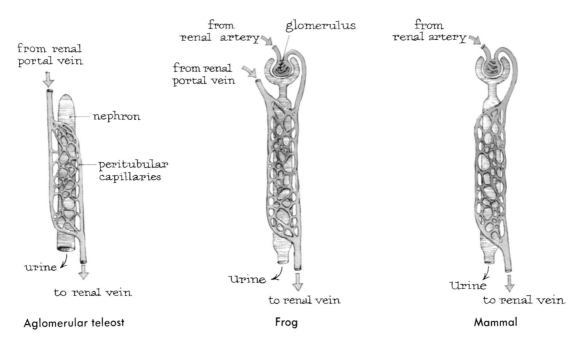

from renal
portal vein

nephron

peritubular
capillaries

urine

to renal vein

Aglomerular teleost

from
renal artery   glomerulus

from renal
portal vein

Urine

to renal vein

Frog

from
renal artery

Urine

to renal vein

Mammal

SCHEMATIC VIEW OF VERTEBRATE NEPHRONS

In the aglomerular marine teleost there is no renal artery, and the nephron is supplied exclusively by venous blood from the renal portal vein. The kidney of the frog is supplied both by the renal artery and the renal portal vein, and the nephron receives both venous and arterial blood. In mammals there is no renal portal vein, and the blood supply to the nephron is exclusively arterial.

It should be noted that these diagrams are much simplified. The nephron, represented as straight and wide, is in reality very slender and intricately coiled. There is apparently some separation of the venous and arterial blood supplies to proximal and distal portions of the nephron in the frog, but as the extent of this separation is uncertain, both arterial and venous blood are here represented as contributing equally to the capillary network.

The entire volume of the extracellular fluid (about eleven quarts in a man weighing one hundred and fifty-five pounds) is filtered through the kidneys some sixteen times each day. This daily filtrate consists of about one hundred seventy-five quarts of water, two-and-a-half pounds of sodium chloride, nearly a pound of sodium bicarbonate, and about one-third of a pound of glucose, together with substantial quantities of potassium, calcium, magnesium, phosphate, sulfate, amino acids, vitamins, and many other substances essential to the body, all of which are carried as solutes in the extracellular fluid. The tubules reabsorb 99 per cent of the water, 95 per cent of the sodium chloride, more than 99 per cent of the sodium bicarbonate and glucose, and similar proportions of the other substances, and transfer them back into the peritubular capillaries. The final product of all this filtering, reabsorption, and tubular excretion is some one-and-a-half quarts of urine, which contains a high concentration of metabolic wastes and other substances present to excess in the blood, and which has a higher concentration of solutes (and, therefore, a higher osmotic pressure) than the blood.

In comparing the kidneys of the frog and the pig, we find a significant difference in the blood supply. The pig's kidney is supplied by blood from only one source: the renal artery. The frog's kidney is supplied by blood from two sources; it receives venous blood from the *renal portal vein* and arterial blood from the *urogenital arteries*. Why is it that the frog's kidney has a double blood supply? Does it serve a functional purpose? If so, what is the reason for the disappearance of the renal portal system in mammals?

There is no general agreement on the answers to these questions in current texts. A possible solution, however, may be suggested by comparing the kidney of the frog with that of certain marine teleosts (bony fishes) in which the glomerulus and renal artery are degenerate or absent. In these fish, venous blood returning via the renal portal vein goes to the peritubular capillaries, and the solutes to be excreted pass into the nephrons by tubular excretion. Very little extracellular fluid filters through the capillary walls into the nephrons because the pressure in the renal portal vein is too low to effect filtration. Such kidneys

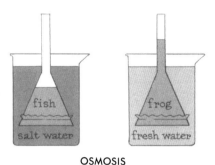

OSMOSIS

If a weak salt solution is separated from a stronger salt solution by a semipermeable membrane, water will pass from the weaker to the stronger solution.

are found in fish which are exclusively marine and never need to excrete excess water. Marine teleosts do not excrete excess water because the concentration of solutes in their internal environment is only about a third that of sea water, and consequently water tends to pass from the fish to the sea by osmosis. The marine fish is constantly working to conserve water. It never has water in excess and passes no more water than necessary as urine.

The frog's problems of water balance are very different from those of the marine teleost because the frog must be able to excrete excess water in an aquatic environment and conserve water on land. The concentration of solutes in the internal environment of the frog is higher than that of fresh water, and consequently water passes into the frog's skin by osmosis. The large subcutaneous lymph spaces under the frog's skin act as reservoirs for excess water, which is pumped into the circulatory system by the lymph hearts.

Blood in the renal artery is under much higher pressure than blood in the renal portal vein. The glomerulus, supplied by blood from the renal artery, acts as a high-pressure filtering device; excess water is filtered off from the blood into the nephrons and eliminated as a very dilute urine. When a frog is submerged, water passes continually through the skin into the subcutaneous lymph spaces by osmosis, and the net uptake of water by the skin is balanced by the formation and elimination of urine.

The frog on land carries a reserve supply of water in the subcutaneous lymph spaces and conserves water by increasing tubular reabsorption and by inhibiting the flow of blood to the glomeruli (thus reducing the rate of glomerular filtration).

In mammals, as in marine teleosts, the main problem is one of water conservation. Water is often scarce on land and what is available must be utilized with a minimum of waste to maintain the proper balance in the internal environment. Since the glomerulus seems to be a device

for getting rid of excess water we might expect mammals, like fish, to have a well-developed renal portal system together with a degenerate or absent glomerulus and renal artery. Instead, we find in mammals *no* renal portal system, and a kidney which produces tremendous amounts of glomerular filtrate only to reabsorb almost all of it back again into the bloodstream. It seems that in the mammalian kidney, the *principle of minimal work* fundamental to so many physiological operations is violated and that we have here an example of extravagant inefficiency. Why is it that so much extracellular fluid is filtered through the glomerulus only to be reabsorbed? Why didn't mammals revert to the apparently more efficient water-conserving kidney of the aglomerular marine teleosts?

The answers to these questions probably have to do with the fact that the most important requirement of the mammalian circulatory system is that it be rapid enough to convey metabolic input and output at the rate required for effective intrinsic temperature control. If a mammal had a renal portal system, the resistance offered to the returning blood by the peritubular capillaries would slow the blood down to an impractically slow rate of flow. Therefore, in mammals, all blood returning from the body bypasses the kidneys and goes directly to the heart. The kidneys are removed from the main line of the venous flow and supplied solely by arterial blood which, because of its high pressure, loses its fluid components by filtration into the nephron, thus making necessary a system of tubular reabsorption to ensure conservation of body fluids.

To sum up: The glomerulus supplied by blood from the renal artery is a high-pressure filtering device which removes fluid from the blood. The nephron without a glomerulus, supplied solely by blood from the renal portal vein, is a low-pressure device which removes wastes by the process of tubular excretion but does not filter much fluid from the blood. Most mammals do not need to excrete large amounts of excess fluid, but the fluid-filtering glomerulus with its associated renal artery is retained in mammals because it offers less resistance to blood flow than the renal portal system offers. Rapid blood circulation is essential for the high metabolic rate of mammals, and the loss of the renal portal system is an example of an anatomical change associated with the evolution of intrinsic temperature control.

It should be understood that this account is much simplified and somewhat speculative. Readers interested in a comprehensive but nontechnical account of the function and evolution of the kidney, with special emphasis on environmental adaptation, should see Homer Smith's admirable book *From Fish to Philosopher* (a Doubleday Anchor paperback).

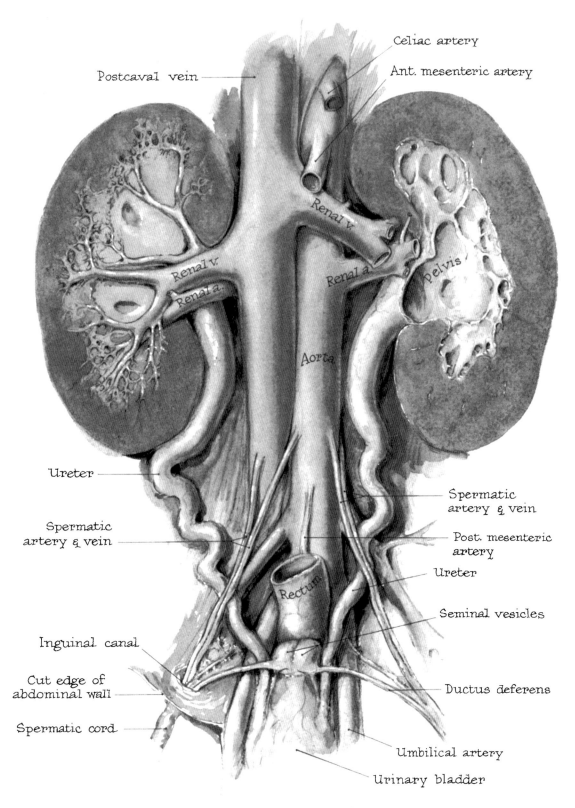

Postcaval vein

Celiac artery

Ant. mesenteric artery

Renal v.

Renal v.

Renal a.

Renal a.

Pelvis

Aorta

Ureter

Spermatic artery & vein

Post. mesenteric artery

Ureter

Spermatic artery & vein

Seminal vesicles

Rectum

Inguinal canal

Cut edge of abdominal wall

Ductus deferens

Spermatic cord

Umbilical artery

Urinary bladder

THE KIDNEYS AND URETERS

The right kidney is dissected to show branches of the renal artery and vein on the ventral side of the renal pelvis. Other branches (not visible from the ventral view) go to the dorsal side of the pelvis. On the left kidney the artery and vein are cut and the ventral pelvic wall is removed to show the inside of the pelvis.

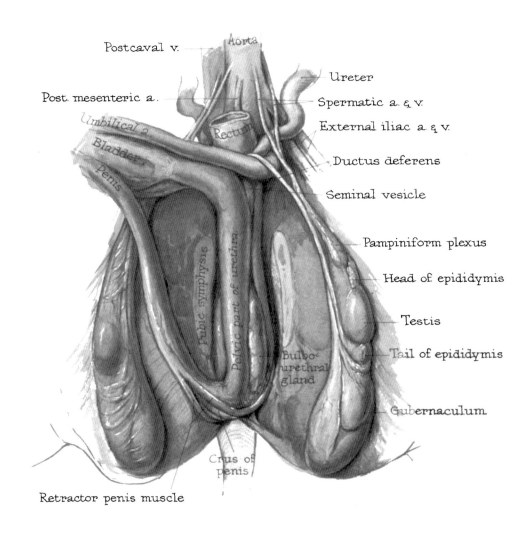

Postcaval v.

Aorta

Ureter

Post. mesenteric a.

Spermatic a. & v.

External iliac a. & v.

Umbilical a.

Rectum

Ductus deferens

Bladder

Seminal vesicle

Penis

Pampiniform plexus

Pubic symphysis

Head of epididymis

Pelvic part of urethra

Testis

Bulbourethral gland

Tail of epididymis

Gubernaculum

Crus of penis

Retractor penis muscle

PELVIC PORTION OF THE MALE UROGENITAL SYSTEM

THE MALE REPRODUCTIVE ORGANS

The sacs containing the *testes* are formed by fascial, muscular, and peritoneal components of the abdominal wall. Cut open the left *scrotal sac* and wash out any coagulated blood which may be found in it. Examine the testis and turn it over to see the *body of the epididymis*, which connects the *head of the epididymis* with the *tail of the epididymis*. Trace the *ductus deferens* to the *seminal vesicles*.

Refer to the lateral views on page 23 to see the relations of the *penis, pubic symphysis, rectum,* and *pelvic portion of the urethra*. Move the penis to one side and probe beneath it to establish the position of the pubic symphysis. Cut the pubic symphysis with a scalpel, being careful not to cut any deeper than necessary. Pull the hindlimbs apart and trim away portions of the pubis on either side as necessary to gain good exposure of the structures illustrated above.

The bulk of each testis consists of *seminiferous tubules,* intricately coiled microscopic ducts within which the *sper-*

matozoa, or male germ cells, are produced. The spermatozoa are stored in the epididymis and pass through the ductus deferens to the urethra. The seminal vesicles and the *bulbo-urethral gland* produce secretions which act as a vehicle for the transport of the spermatozoa, and the term *semen* is applied to these secretions plus the spermatozoa. The *prostate gland* also contributes a secretion to the semen. It is a small gland lying between the lobes of the seminal vesicles near the junction of the bladder and the pelvic portion of the urethra. Because of its immature condition it is not readily identified in the fetal pig.

In addition to producing spermatozoa, the testes secrete hormones termed *androgens* which affect sexual development and behavior and influence metabolism. The production of these hormones is interrelated with the hypophysial hormones, which initiate spermatogenesis and the secretion of androgens.

In the pig, as in the frog, the embryonic testes originate behind the peritoneum near the kidneys. During fetal development, the testes of the pig move posteriorly behind the peritoneum and descend into the *scrotum*, carrying with them the spermatic vessels, ductus deferens, nerves, and lymphatics which constitute the *spermatic cord*. Before its descent, the testis is connected to the scrotum by a band of tissue termed the *gubernaculum*, and it is thought that this structure is functional in effecting the descent of the testes into the scrotum.

In all cold-blooded vertebrates and in some mammals (elephants, whales, and others), the testes remain permanently within the body cavity. In other mammals, they descend into the scrotum only during periods of sexual activity; in primates and many others, they remain in the scrotum permanently. This displacement of the testes is connected with the fact that in many mammals the spermatozoa are unable to develop at mammalian body temperatures. In such animals, the testes are carried in the scrotum, which apparently affords a cooler and more favorable temperature. If the testes of an animal with a scrotum are moved back into the body cavity, no spermatozoa are produced. Anomalous individuals in which the testes do not complete their descent into the scrotum are invariably sterile, but if the testes are surgically moved from the body cavity into the scrotum, viable spermatozoa are often produced. It is not understood why the high mammalian body temperature necessary for the development of the ova and the embryo is not also favorable for the development of the spermatozoa.

In comparing sperm transport in the frog and the pig, we find evidence of the evolutionary struggle between the kidneys and the gonads for control of the *Wolffian duct*, or primitive excretory duct of the kidney. In frogs, the Wolffian duct serves for the transport of both spermatozoa and urine, but in mammals it is monopolized by the testes and termed the *ductus deferens*. The mammalian kidney has formed a new excretory duct, the *ureter*, which has no homolog in the frog.

In the frog, numerous minute ducts, the *vasa efferentia*, carry spermatozoa from the testis through the kidney to the Wolffian duct. The vasa efferentia originate embryologically from the renal corpuscles and in some frogs this connection persists in the adult, so that the spermatozoa pass through the nephrons on their way to the Wolffian duct.

The mammalian homolog of the anterior part of the frog's kidney is the *epididymis*, and the tubules of the epididymis are the homologs of the nephrons through which the frog's spermatozoa pass to reach the Wolffian duct. The ductus deferens of the pig corresponds to the Wolffian duct of the frog, and the renal portal vein is represented in the pig by the *pampiniform plexus*, a network of veins on the ductus deferens. Even the kidneys of the frog and the pig are not strictly homologous. The adult mammalian kidney arises only from the posterior portion of the embryonic kidney, whereas the frog's kidney arises from the entire length of the embryonic kidney.

THE FEMALE REPRODUCTIVE ORGANS

Refer to the lateral views on page 22 to see the relations of the *pubic symphysis, urethra, vagina,* and *rectum.* Probe in the midline to establish the position of the pubic symphysis and cut it with a scalpel, being careful not to cut deeper than necessary. Pull the hindlimbs apart and trim away portions of the pubis on either side to gain a good exposure of the structures illustrated on the opposite page. Dissect the pelvic portion of the urethra away from the vagina and establish the point at which the urethra enters the *urogenital sinus.* Cut the *bladder, umbilical arteries,* and left *ureter* to make a dissection resembling the illustration on the opposite page.

Cut the *broad ligament* which attaches the *uterine horns* to the dorsal body wall and remove the *uterus, vagina,* and *urogenital sinus.* Insert the point of your scissors in the *urogenital orifice,* make a cut along the dorsal side of the urogenital tract, and pin it out flat in a dissecting pan. Identify the structures illustrated in Fig. *B,* opposite.

Mammalian eggs, or *ova,* develop within the *ovary.* Mature ova lie within fluid-filled capsules, the *ovarian follicles,* near the surface of the ovary. At intervals the follicles containing the ova rupture and the ova pass into the abdominal cavity; this process is termed *ovulation.* The ova enter the *abdominal ostium of the Fallopian tube* and are carried down the tube by peristaltic movements. If spermatozoa are present in the female genital tract, fertilization may occur (normally in the Fallopian tube) and the fertilized egg, or *zygote,* passes into the uterine horn, where fetal development takes place.

The frequency of ovulation and the number of ova released varies considerably in various mammalian species. In the dog, ovulation occurs every six months; in humans, every 28 days; in rats, every five days.

In addition to producing ova, the ovaries secrete two kinds of hormones, *estrogens* and *progesterone,* which affect female sexual development and behavior. The interaction of ovarian hormones with hormones produced in the hypophysis regulates the estrus and menstrual cycles.

Mammals exhibit a number of adaptations designed to ensure a stable environment for the sexual products and the fetus. The external genitalia of the male and the vagina of the female ensure internal fertilization, and the uterus provides a protective compartment for the development of the fetus. All chemical exchanges between the mammalian fetus and the external environment are mediated through the maternal circulation. The placenta represents an adaptation for the exchange of respiratory gases, nutriment, and metabolic wastes between the fetal and maternal blood.

The frog's egg, in contrast, is fertilized outside the maternal body. The developing tadpole carries on respiratory exchange with the surrounding water and obtains nutriment from the yolk of the egg. Within several weeks it breaks out of the gelatinous covering of the egg and is ready to feed itself.

The warm-blooded mode of life makes it impossible for a mammalian fetus to develop outside the maternal body. Even if it were supplied with large quantities of nutriment in the form of yolk, it could not survive the thermal conditions in which tadpoles thrive. So much heat would be dissipated through the relatively large body surface that the warm-blooded embryo could not possibly maintain its own temperature at the required level.

The tadpole depends for survival on temperate weather. Frogs, therefore, ovulate only once a year, in the late winter or early spring, thus ensuring the young of birth at a favorable season and the chance to mature before winter. The number of eggs released during ovulation in the frog varies with the species, but may be as great as twenty thousand. The eggs break through the ovarian follicles and are carried by the action of peritoneal cilia to the funnel-shaped mouths of the oviducts, which are located in the anterior part of the body cavity at the base of the lungs. The eggs pass single-file down the oviducts, within which they receive protective coats of jelly. Then they enter the ovisacs, where they are retained until ovulation is complete.

During ovulation the male clings to the back of the female, and when the eggs are extruded from the cloaca the male discharges his spermatic fluid over them and fertilization occurs in the water. In frogs, we find neither

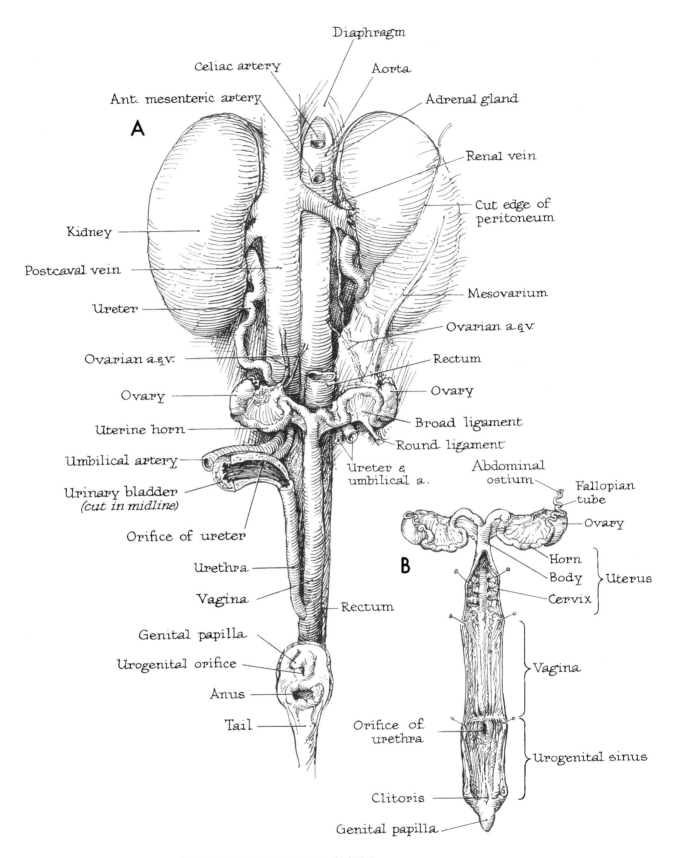

Diaphragm

Celiac artery

Aorta

Ant. mesenteric artery

Adrenal gland

A

Renal vein

Cut edge of peritoneum

Kidney

Postcaval vein

Mesovarium

Ureter

Ovarian a. & v.

Ovarian a. & v.

Rectum

Ovary

Ovary

Uterine horn

Broad ligament

Round ligament

Umbilical artery

Ureter & umbilical a.

Abdominal ostium

Fallopian tube

Urinary bladder (cut in midline)

Ovary

B

Horn

Body

Cervix

} Uterus

Orifice of ureter

Urethra

Vagina

Rectum

Vagina

Genital papilla

Urogenital orifice

Orifice of urethra

Anus

Urogenital sinus

Tail

Clitoris

Genital papilla

THE FEMALE UROGENITAL SYSTEM

41

the external genitalia nor the vagina characteristic of mammals.* The spermatozoa, eggs, urine, and feces all pass to the exterior via a common chamber, the cloaca.

Examine a pregnant uterus and compare it with the fetal uterus. Make a cut in the wall of one of the uterine horns and observe the folds of the *uterine mucosa* (inner layer of the uterine wall) and the convoluted surface of the *chorion*. These folds serve to increase the surfaces across which the exchange of metabolic products occurs. Both the chorion and the uterine mucosa are richly supplied with blood vessels, but the fetal blood does not mix with the maternal blood. The two bloodstreams are separated by a membrane which allows the exchange of small molecules, but not of blood proteins or corpuscles.

* There are exceptions to this, as there are to most generalizations. Noble tells us: "The ovoviparous frogs of Africa, *Nectophrynoides*, practice internal fertilization, although no external organs for transferring the sperm are known in these frogs. In the 'tailed' frog of America, *Ascaphus*, the 'tail,' an extension of the cloaca, serves as an intromittent organ."

The term *placenta* is applied to the structures which effect the exchange of metabolic materials between the fetus and the mother. In the pig the placenta consists of the chorion and the uterine mucosa.

Open the chorion and expose the fetuses. Each fetus is surrounded by a transparent membrane termed the *amnion*. The blood vessels seen on the inner surface of the chorion actually lie within the *allantois*, a thin membrane fused with the chorion. Open the amnion and identify the *umbilical cord*. Observe that the umbilical cord attaches the fetus to the fetal membranes but not to the uterus.

The adaptations which made it possible for eggs and embryos to survive in a nonaquatic environment were of primary importance for the evolution of terrestrial life. An excellent treatment of this topic will be found in A. A. Romer's article, "Origin of the Amniote Egg," in *Science Monthly* (1957), 85:57–63.

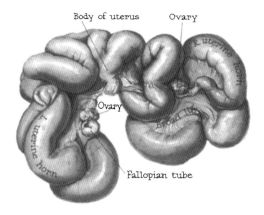

THE MATURE UTERUS

Dorsal view of a pregnant uterus removed a few weeks before the middle of the gestation period.

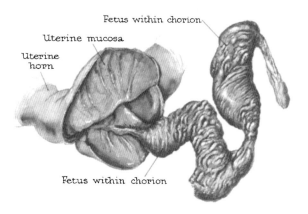

One of the uterine horns is opened and the chorion surrounding two fetuses is pulled out. Respiratory and nutritive exchange takes place between the chorion and the uterine mucosa, which together constitute the placenta.

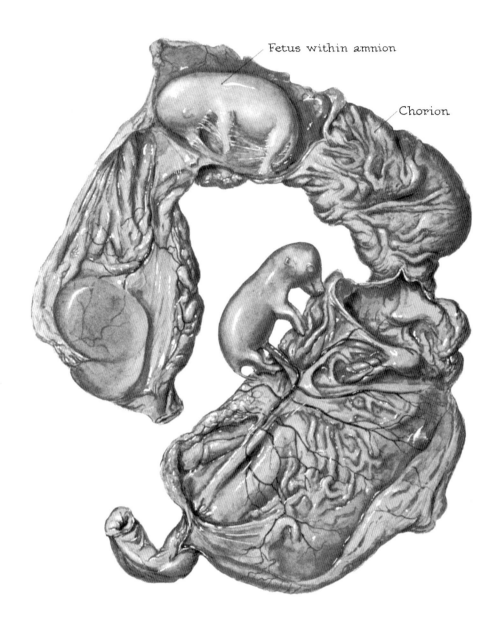

Fetus within amnion

Chorion

THE FETAL MEMBRANES

The chorion is opened to reveal two fetuses. The blood vessels seen here lie within the allantois, a thin membrane fused with the inner surface of the chorion.

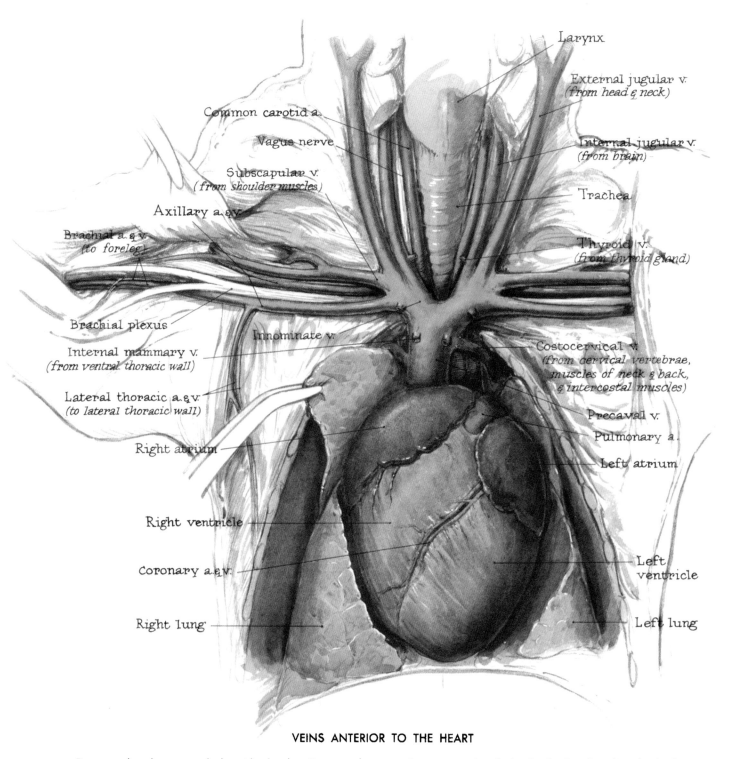

Larynx

External jugular v.
(from head & neck)

Common carotid a.

Vagus nerve

Internal jugular v.
(from brain)

Subscapular v.
(from shoulder muscles)

Trachea

Axillary a. & v.

Brachial a. & v.
(to foreleg)

Thyroid v.
(from thyroid gland)

Brachial plexus

Innominate v.

Costocervical v.
(from cervical vertebrae,
muscles of neck & back,
& intercostal muscles)

Internal mammary v.
(from ventral thoracic wall)

Lateral thoracic a. & v.
(to lateral thoracic wall)

Precaval v.

Pulmonary a.

Right atrium

Left atrium

Right ventricle

Left
ventricle

Coronary a. & v.

Right lung

Left lung

VEINS ANTERIOR TO THE HEART

Remove the thymus and thyroid glands. Remove the sternocephalicus, superficial pectoral, anterior deep pectoral, and posterior deep pectoral muscles. Trim away the *pericardium* (the membranous sac enclosing the heart) and the thoracic portion of the thymus gland, and cut the rib cage as necessary to gain good exposure of the heart and vessels. Using forceps and fine scissors, clean away the fat and connective tissue to expose the vessels illustrated above.

The arrangement of the veins is variable and it may help to keep this general plan in mind. There are four major areas to be drained: the head and neck, the brain, the forelimb, and the shoulder. These areas are drained by four large veins which will be found in almost all specimens: the *external jugular*, *internal jugular*, *brachial*, and *subscapular veins*. The blood from these veins must be collected into one channel to enter the *right atrium*, and it is in the manner of this connection that many variations occur. The subscapular and brachial veins often join to form a *subclavian vein* before entering the *innominate vein*, and small veins from the lateral and dorsal muscles of the thorax may be variable in number and position.

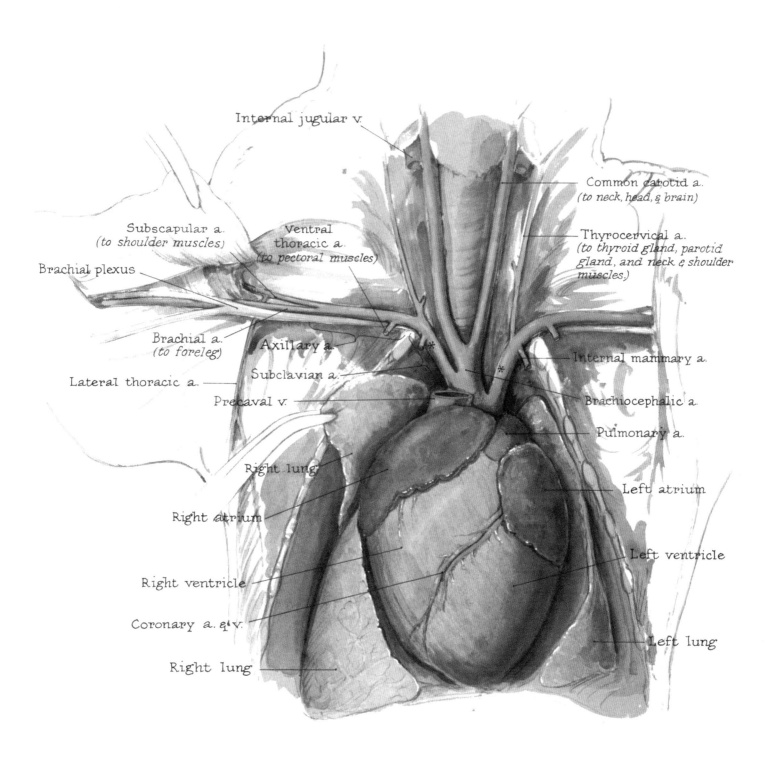

Internal jugular v.

Common carotid a.
(to neck, head, & brain)

Subscapular a.
(to shoulder muscles)

Ventral
thoracic a.
(to pectoral muscles)

Thyrocervical a.
(to thyroid gland, parotid
gland, and neck & shoulder
muscles.)

Brachial plexus

Brachial a.
(to foreleg)

Axillary a.

Internal mammary a.

Lateral thoracic a.

Subclavian a.

Brachiocephalic a.

Precaval v.

Pulmonary a.

Right lung

Left atrium

Right atrium

Right ventricle

Left ventricle

Coronary a. & v.

Left lung

Right lung

ARTERIES ANTERIOR TO THE HEART

Remove the veins and identify the arteries illustrated above. At the points indicated by asterisks, the *costocervical arteries* (not visible from the ventral view) branch dorsally from the subclavian. This is illustrated in the lateral view on page 46. At the level of the larynx, the *common carotid arteries* divide into *external carotids* (to jaw muscles, tongue, and face) and *internal carotids* (to brain).

The instructor shoud select certain students to leave the veins anterior to the heart intact and make a demonstration dissection similar to the lateral view on page 46. He may also wish to select a specimen with an injected portal vein and make a demonstration dissection similar to the lateral view on page 47.

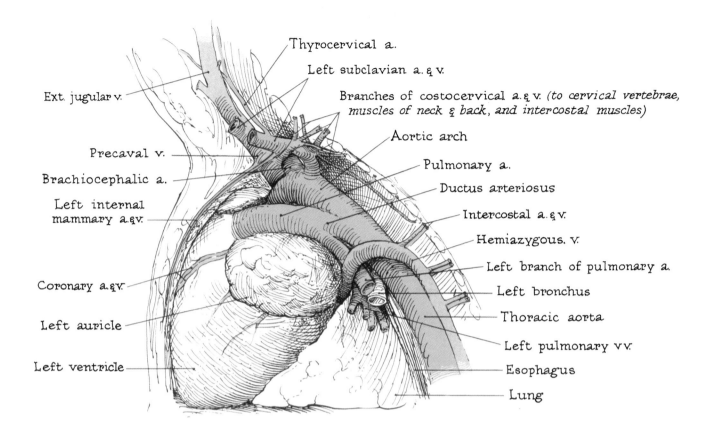

Thyrocervical a.

Left subclavian a. & v.

Branches of costocervical a. & v. *(to cervical vertebrae, muscles of neck & back, and intercostal muscles)*

Ext. jugular v.

Aortic arch

Pulmonary a.

Precaval v.

Ductus arteriosus

Brachiocephalic a.

Intercostal a. & v.

Left internal mammary a. & v.

Hemiazygous. v.

Left branch of pulmonary a.

Left bronchus

Coronary a. & v.

Thoracic aorta

Left auricle

Left pulmonary v v.

Left ventricle

Esophagus

Lung

LATERAL VIEW OF THE HEART

The left lung and the left side of the thorax are removed
to reveal the heart.

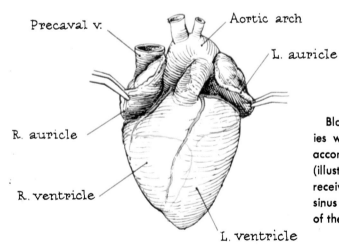

Precaval v.

Aortic arch

L. auricle

R. auricle

R. ventricle

L. ventricle

THE CORONARY ARTERIES

Blood is supplied to the heart muscle by coronary arteries which originate at the base of the aorta. The veins accompanying these arteries return to the coronary sinus (illustrated in the dorsal view of the heart), which also receives blood from the hemiazygous vein. The coronary sinus enters the right atrium just caudal to the entrance of the postcaval vein.

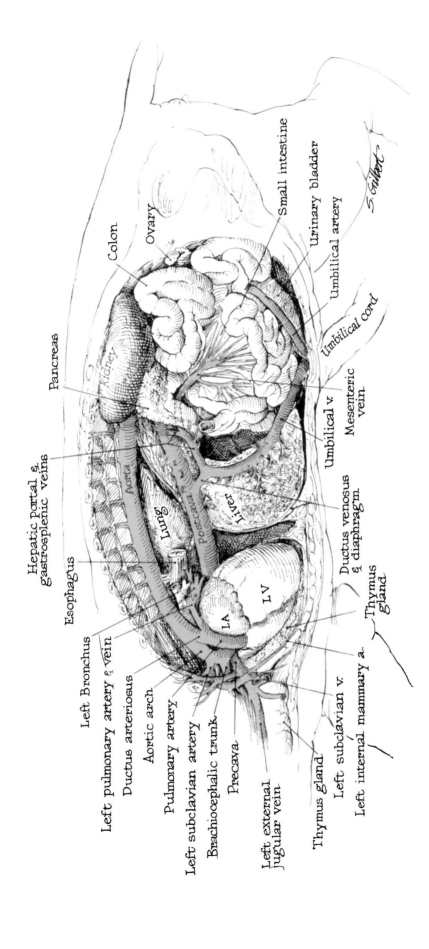

Hepatic Portal &
gastrosplenic veins

Esophagus

Left Bronchus

Ductus arteriosus

Aortic arch

Pulmonary artery

Left subclavian artery

Brachiocephalic trunk

Precava

Left external
jugular vein

Thymus gland

Left subclavian v.

Left internal mammary a.

Left pulmonary artery & vein

Pancreas

Colon

Ovary

Small intestine

Urinary bladder

Umbilical artery

Umbilical cord

Mesenteric
vein

Umbilical v.

Ductus venosus
& diaphragm.

Thymus
gland

Kidney

Aorta

Lung

Postcava

Liver

LA

LV

THE PORTAL VEIN

The liver is cut in the midline and the stomach is removed to show the course of the umbilical and portal veins. The small intestine is retracted and the mesentery is partially dissected to show the origin of the mesenteric vein. Many arteries are accompanied by veins of the same name. However, there are no veins entering the postcaval vein which correspond to the celiac, anterior mesenteric, and posterior mesenteric arteries of the aorta. In the adult portal system, these arteries supply the abdominal viscera with blood which passes through the capillaries of the digestive tube, enters the liver via the portal vein, and again passes through a system of capillaries (the sinusoids of the liver) before entering the postcaval vein through the hepatic veins. The ductus venosus and umbilical vein are fetal structures which close after birth.

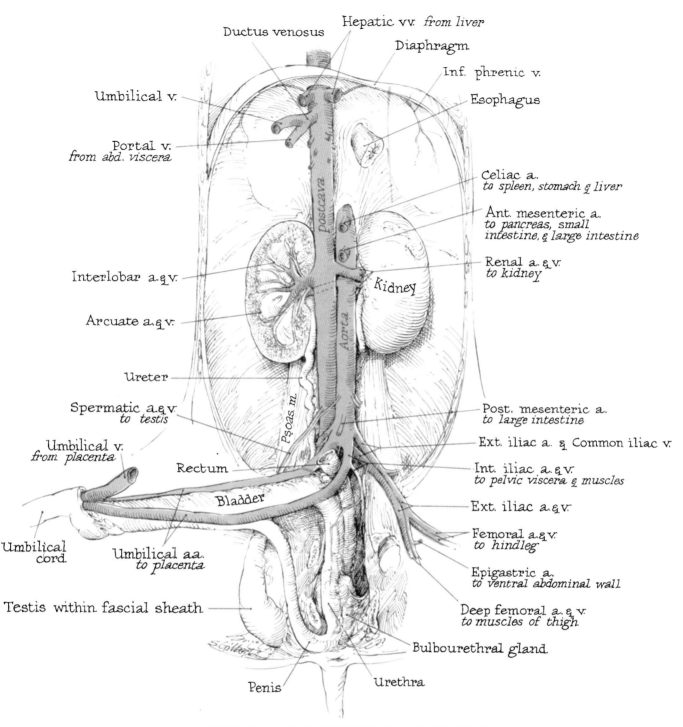

Ductus venosus

Hepatic vv. *from liver*

Diaphragm

Inf. phrenic v.

Umbilical v.

Esophagus

Portal v.
from abd. viscera

Celiac a.
to spleen, stomach & liver

Ant. mesenteric a.
*to pancreas, small
intestine, & large intestine*

Renal a. & v.
to kidney

postcava

Interlobar a. & v.

Kidney

Arcuate a. & v.

Aorta

Ureter

Psoas m.

Post. mesenteric a.
to large intestine

Spermatic a. & v.
to testis

Ext. iliac a. & Common iliac v.

Int. iliac a. & v.
to pelvic viscera & muscles

Umbilical v.
from placenta

Rectum

Bladder

Ext. iliac a. & v.

Femoral a. & v.
to hindleg

Umbilical
cord

Umbilical aa.
to placenta

Epigastric a.
to ventral abdominal wall

Testis within fascial sheath

Deep femoral a. & v.
to muscles of thigh

Bulbourethral gland

Penis

Urethra

ARTERIES AND VEINS POSTERIOR TO THE DIAPHRAGM

Use fine scissors and forceps to remove the peritoneum and connective tissue from the abdominal vessels. Identify the structures illustrated above. Observe the mass of tough white tissue which surrounds the origins of celiac and anterior mesenteric arteries. This is the celiac plexus, part of the autonomic nervous system.

Six pairs of *lumbar arteries* (not visible from the ventral view) arise from the dorsal side of the aorta to supply the muscles of the back. The lumbar arteries are accompanied by six pairs of *lumbar veins* which enter the dorsal side of the *postcaval vein.*

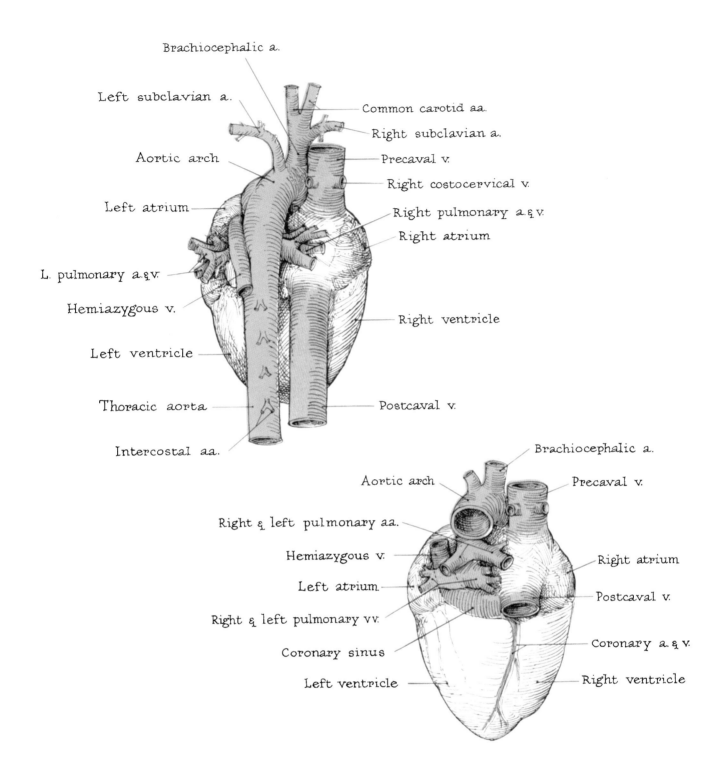

Brachiocephalic a.

Left subclavian a.

Aortic arch

Left atrium

L. pulmonary a.&v.

Hemiazygous v.

Left ventricle

Thoracic aorta

Intercostal aa.

Common carotid aa.

Right subclavian a.

Precaval v.

Right costocervical v.

Right pulmonary a.&v.

Right atrium

Right ventricle

Postcaval v.

Brachiocephalic a.

Aortic arch

Right & left pulmonary aa.

Hemiazygous v.

Left atrium

Right & left pulmonary vv.

Coronary sinus

Left ventricle

Precaval v.

Right atrium

Postcaval v.

Coronary a.&v.

Right ventricle

DORSAL VIEWS OF THE HEART

Cut the common carotid and *left subclavian arteries* as indicated above. Pick away portions of the lung as necessary to expose portions of the *hemiazygos vein*, the *thoracic aorta,* and the *postcaval vein*. Pull the top of the heart away from the lungs, identifying and cutting the pulmonary vessels, postcaval vein, and thoracic aorta to remove the heart.

Blood from the *intercostal veins* is returned by the hemiazygos vein through the *coronary sinus* to the right atrium. Above, the hemiazygos vein is seen arching over the left pulmonary vessels. Below, dotted lines indicate its path behind the pulmonary vessels. In some specimens, the hemiazygos vein may enter the right atrium or the postcaval vein.

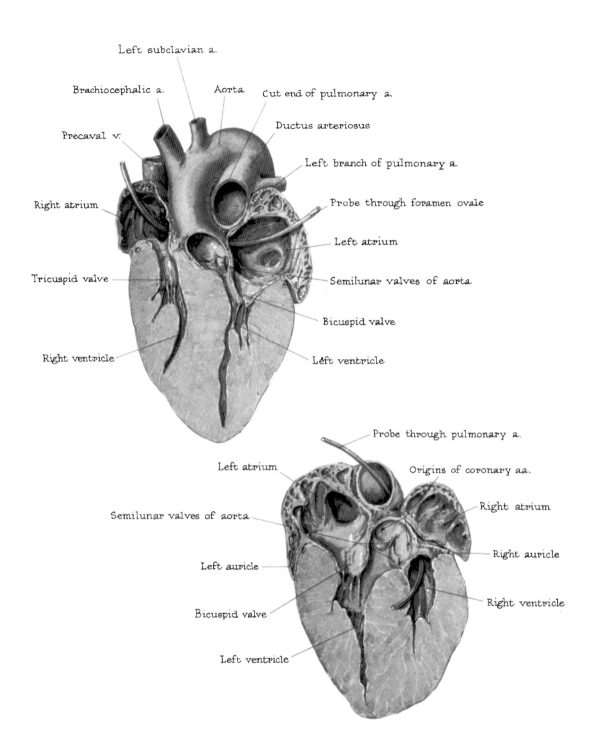

Left subclavian a.

Brachiocephalic a.   Aorta   Cut end of pulmonary a.

Precaval v.   Ductus arteriosus

Left branch of pulmonary a.

Right atrium   Probe through foramen ovale

Left atrium

Tricuspid valve   Semilunar valves of aorta

Bicuspid valve

Right ventricle   Left ventricle

Probe through pulmonary a.

Left atrium   Origins of coronary aa.

Right atrium

Semilunar valves of aorta

Right auricle

Left auricle

Bicuspid valve   Right ventricle

Left ventricle

INTERIOR VIEWS OF THE HEART

Use razor blade and scissors to make a vertical section of the heart in the coronal plane. Cut as much as possible with the razor blade; scissors will be necessary only for severing the masses of injected latex. Wash out the coagulated blood and the latex from the interior of the heart. Pass probes through the *foramen ovale* and the *pulmonary artery* and identify the structures illustrated.

Mature beef hearts will be provided for comparison with the fetal heart. Trim away the pericardium and fat from the beef heart as necessary to identify the structures illustrated in the dorsal and ventral views on the opposite page. Then cut away portions of the right lateral heart wall to expose the right atrium and ventricle as illustrated. Similarly, cut away portions of the left atrium and ventricle on the opposite side.

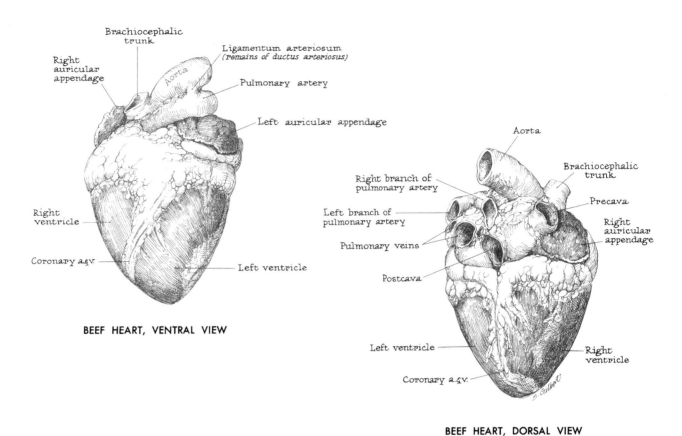

BEEF HEART, VENTRAL VIEW

Brachiocephalic trunk

Right auricular appendage

Ligamentum arteriosum
(remains of ductus arteriosus)

Pulmonary artery

Left auricular appendage

Aorta

Right ventricle

Coronary a.&v.

Left ventricle

BEEF HEART, DORSAL VIEW

Aorta

Right branch of pulmonary artery

Brachiocephalic trunk

Precava

Left branch of pulmonary artery

Pulmonary veins

Right auricular appendage

Postcava

Left ventricle

Right ventricle

Coronary a.&v.

S. Gilbert

RIGHT LATERAL VIEW

Wall of right auricular appendage

Aorta

Brachiocephalic trunk

Pulmonary artery

Opening of precava into right atrium

Pulmonary semilunar valve

Opening of postcava into right atrium

Opening of coronary sinus

Trabeculae carneae

Tricuspid valve (medial cusp)

Right ventricle

Chordae tendineae

Papillary muscle

LEFT LATERAL VIEW

Aorta

Wall of left auricular appendage

Brachiocephalic trunk

Opening of pulmonary vein into left atrium

Opening of right coronary artery

Aortic semilunar valve

Bicuspid valve (posterior cusp)

Chordae tendineae

Left ventricle

Papillary muscle

Trabeculae carneae

S. Gilbert

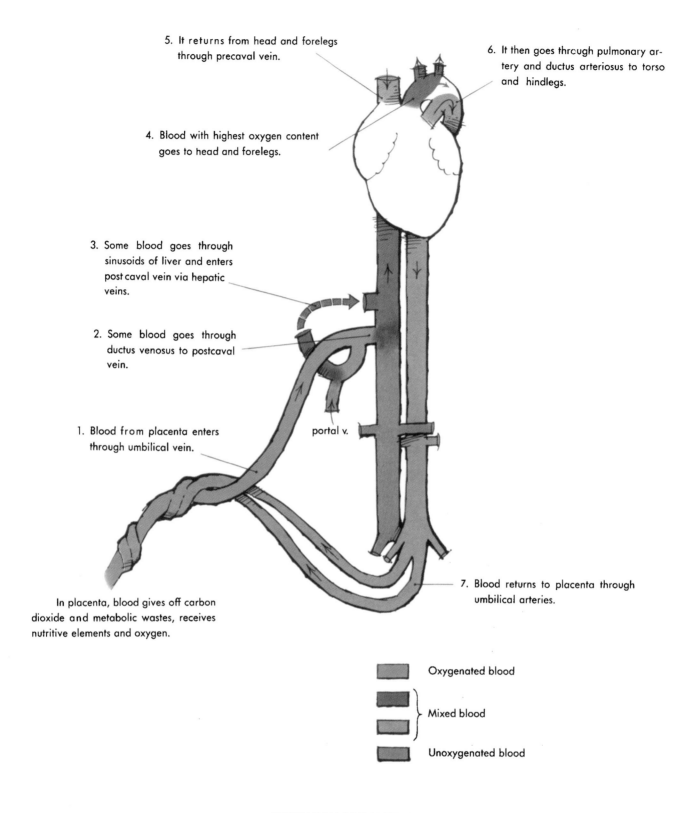

5. It returns from head and forelegs through precaval vein.

6. It then goes through pulmonary artery and ductus arteriosus to torso and hindlegs.

4. Blood with highest oxygen content goes to head and forelegs.

3. Some blood goes through sinusoids of liver and enters post caval vein via hepatic veins.

2. Some blood goes through ductus venosus to postcaval vein.

portal v.

1. Blood from placenta enters through umbilical vein.

7. Blood returns to placenta through umbilical arteries.

In placenta, blood gives off carbon dioxide and metabolic wastes, receives nutritive elements and oxygen.

Oxygenated blood

} Mixed blood

Unoxygenated blood

CIRCULATION IN THE FETUS

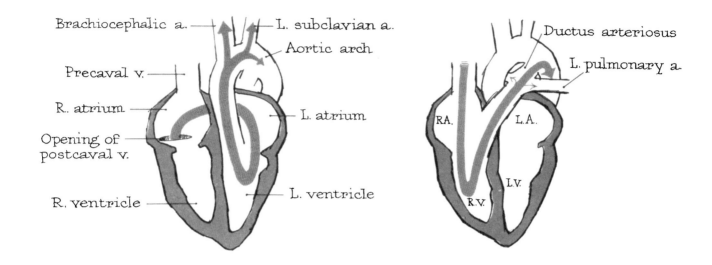

Brachiocephalic a.

L. subclavian a.

Aortic arch

Precaval v.

R. atrium

L. atrium

Opening of
postcaval v.

R. ventricle

L. ventricle

Ductus arteriosus

L. pulmonary a.

RA.

L.A.

L.V.

R.V.

CIRCULATION IN THE FETAL HEART

Blood of relatively high oxygen content enters the right atrium from the postcaval vein. It goes through the foramen ovale into the left atrium. From the left atrium it goes to the left ventricle, and from the left ventricle to the aorta to supply the head and forelimbs.

Blood of relatively lower oxygen content returns from the head and forelimbs via the precaval vein to the right atrium. From the right atrium it goes to the right ventricle, then through the pulmonary artery and the ductus arteriosus into the aorta.

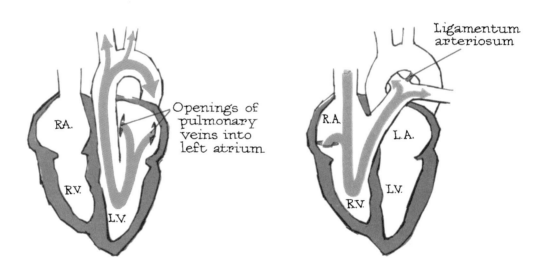

RA.

R.V.

L.V.

Openings of
pulmonary
veins into
left atrium

Ligamentum
arteriosum

R.A.

L.A.

L.V.

R.V.

CIRCULATION IN THE ADULT HEART

Oxygenated blood enters the left atrium via the pulmonary veins. It goes to the left ventricle, and from the left ventricle to the body.

Unoxygenated blood enters the right atrium from the precaval and postcaval veins. It goes to the right ventricle,

and from the right ventricle to the lungs via the pulmonary arteries. The ductus arteriosus is obliterated; its remains appear as a band of fibrous tissue termed the *ligamentum arteriosum*.

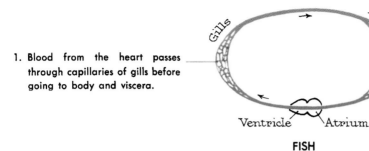

1. Blood from the heart passes through capillaries of gills before going to body and viscera.

2. Blood going to body passes through one set of capillaries, and blood going to renal or hepatic portal systems passes through two sets of capillaries before returning to heart.

FISH

2. Blood richest in oxygen goes directly to body and viscera.

1. Blood poorest in oxygen goes to lungs, skin, and mucous membrane of mouth.

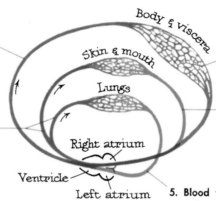

3. Blood going to body passes through one set of capillaries, and blood going to renal or hepatic portal systems passes through two sets of capillaries before returning to heart.

4. Blood from skin and mucous membrane of mouth mixes with venous blood from body and is returned to right atrium.

5. Blood from lungs returns to left atrium. Some mixing of oxygenated and unoxygenated blood occurs in ventricle.

FROG

2. It then returns to heart, from which it goes directly to body and viscera.

1. Unoxygenated blood from heart passes through capillaries of lungs.

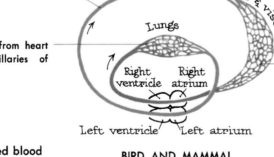

3. Blood going to body passes through one set of capillaries, and blood going to hepatic portal system passes through two sets of capillaries. There is no renal portal system.

Oxygenated blood

Mixed blood

Unoxygenated blood

BIRD AND MAMMAL

DIAGRAMS OF VERTEBRATE CIRCULATORY SYSTEMS

Because of their greater activity, most terrestrial vertebrates have a higher metabolic rate than cold-blooded aquatic vertebrates. This has been achieved by a reduction in the number of capillary nets through which the blood passes before returning to the heart and also by the development of a double circuit in the heart to pump oxygenated blood directly to the body and viscera. The frog is descended from a vertebrate ancestor representing an intermediate stage in this development.

THE CIRCULATORY SYSTEM

Study the diagrams on pages 52, 53, and 54. Be able to describe the circulation in a typical fish, frog, and mammal, and to describe the difference between the fetal and adult circulations in the mammal. You should also be able to identify the structures found in the fetal and adult mammalian hearts and to account for the relations of the valves and vessels in terms of blood flow.

In comparing the heart of the pig with that of the frog, we find a number of major changes. The aortic arch of the pig is the homolog of the left systemic arch of the frog, whereas the frog's right systemic arch has no homolog in the pig. The base of the aortic arch and the main trunk of the pulmonary arches as seen in the pig are homologs of the single main arterial channel (*bulbus cordis* and *truncus arteriosus*) which carries both oxygenated and unoxygenated blood from the single ventricle of the frog.

The heart of the frog is sometimes referred to as "a transitional stage in the evolution of the double-pump heart," a statement which may produce the erroneous impression that mammals had ancestors with hearts anatomically similar to the modern frog heart. Actually, modern amphibians exhibit many specializations which probably depart widely from the transitional stages in the main line of vertebrate descent. Whether the divided atrium evolved before the divided ventricle is a matter of conjecture. The specializations for partially separating the oxygenated and unoxygenated bloodstreams and the circulatory adaptations connected with cutaneous respiration and hibernation are probably not primitive characteristics.*

If the heart of the frog may not be regarded as a transitional evolutionary stage, it is at least tempting to see the evolution of the double-pump circulation as a trend toward increased circulatory efficiency. In describing the amphibian circulatory system, A. S. Romer writes: "With the introduction of the lung circuit into the circulatory system and the abolition in adult amphibians of gill breathing, circulatory efficiency is greatly promoted. The gill capillary system is eliminated; hence all body tissues are reached arterially directly with little loss of pressure."

Other writers describe the circulation of amphibians as *less* efficient than that of fish. John A. Moore, for instance, writes:

> The change to land living, with its associated loss of gill respiration and the beginning of lung respiration, changed the route of circulation. Blood now passes the heart twice in making a complete circuit of lungs and tissues, and arterial and venous blood are mixed. Physiologically speaking this is less efficient than the unmixed blood of the fish. It was a great advance in evolution for the amphibia to invade the land, but one of the penalties was this less efficient circulatory system.†

If it is true that the extent to which oxygenated blood and unoxygenated blood mix is a criterion of circulatory efficiency, we are faced with the paradox that although the circulation of the adult mammal is more efficient than the circulation of the frog, the circulation of the tadpole is more efficient than the circulation of the mammalian fetus. While the tadpole breathes by means of gills, its circulation is functionally similar to that of the fish. In the mammalian fetus, oxygenated blood from the placenta mixes with unoxygenated blood in the postcaval vein and none of the tissues receive pure oxygenated blood.

Quantitative measurements of the extent to which oxygenated and unoxygenated blood actually mix in the amphibian ventricle show that in some cases there is very little mixing. De Graaf reports that in the toad, *Xenopus laevis*, "the body and the head receive the most highly oxygenated blood, only scarcely contaminated with oxygen-poor blood." He concludes that "the oxygen needs of *Xenopus* may at times be extremely low," and that "the blood contains more oxygen than is required in many circumstances."

In a summary of recent work on amphibian circulation Foxon writes: ". . . as the respiratory methods of the amphibians are varied so are the circulatory methods and it is impossible to speak of a generalized scheme for the mode of action of the 'amphibian' heart." He concludes that ". . . the circulation of the blood from the heart is carried out in different amphibians in very varied ways; these appear to be well adapted to the physiological needs of the animals."

The speed of circulation, blood volume, oxygen-carrying capacity of the blood, total capillary surface, and the

---

*A discussion of this topic will be found in chapter 3, "Blood and Respiration," by G. E. H. Foxon in *The Physiology of the Amphibia*, ed. John A. Moore (New York: Academic Press, 1964).

†John A. Moore, *Principles of Zoology* (New York: Oxford University Press, 1957).

form of the heart and vessels are mutually interdependent variables which show a great variety of adaptations in response to different environmental demands in amphibians as well as in other vertebrates. No meaningful assessment of circulatory efficiency can be made without taking into account the total picture presented by the integrated action of these factors. Attempts to do so are misleading in that they obscure the functional interrelationships between the organism and the environment.

The evolution of the double-pump circulation in mammals and birds is connected with the development of intrinsic temperature control and with the fact that moving on land or in the air requires a greater expenditure of muscular effort than moving in water. A fish consumes a relatively small amount of oxygen while at rest and requires three or four times more oxygen when swimming rapidly. Man, on the other hand, has a relatively high metabolic rate while at rest and consumes fifteen to twenty times more oxygen when running at a speed comparable to that of the swimming fish. Still higher rates of oxygen consumption occur in birds. A flying pigeon consumes thirty times as much oxygen as a resting pigeon. (The greatest increase is found in insects, which may consume fifty to two hundred times as much oxygen in flight as they do at rest.)

The fish has a relatively slow heart rate, low blood pressure, small blood volume, and small total area of capillary surface. The relatively rapid heart, high blood pressure, large blood volume, and large capillary surface of mammals are adaptations connected with a higher metabolic rate and increased activity.

The simultaneous development of increased capillary surface and rapid heart rate creates a problem in hydraulics, for the greater capillary surface offers more resistance to the flow of blood, with the result that the work of the heart is increased by two factors at once; it must beat faster and at the same time it must overcome increased capillary resistance due to friction.

In the circulatory systems of terrestrial vertebrates, this problem is met by reducing the number of capillary networks through which the blood passes in a single circuit. No terrestrial vertebrate retains the fishlike circulation in which blood passes through at least two and often three capillary systems before returning to the heart. In the frog, much of the blood bypasses the lungs and goes directly to the body. The lungs and respiratory skin surface are supplied by blood diverted from the main stream and shunted around a short supplementary circuit. In mammals and birds, a separate atrium and ventricle supply the pulmonary circuit, while the resistance offered by

the renal capillaries is circumvented by a mechanism similar in principle to that of the frog's respiratory circuit: blood destined for the kidneys is diverted from the main stream and shunted around a short supplementary circuit, and the renal portal system is abandoned.

Although it is true that the evolutionary trend is toward a reduction in the *number* of capillary networks through which blood passes in a single circuit, this cannot in itself be interpreted as a measure of increased efficiency. Most blood leaving the ventricle of the mammal passes through only one capillary network before returning to the heart, but that single capillary network may have a relatively greater total surface (and therefore offer greater resistance to blood flow) than all three capillary networks through which the blood of the fish passes in a single circuit.

Any meaningful statement about the relative efficiency of circulatory systems must be made in terms of quantitative measurements of the cost of blood production and transport (taking into account the fact that this cost is one of many mutually interdependent physiological variables). Attempts to determine the exact cost in energy of blood production and transport are necessarily approximate because of the many variables involved, but estimates suggest that the cost of blood is comparable to that of other active body tissues, and there is no evidence to indicate that the frog spends a disproportionately large fraction of its total energy output on the production and circulation of blood.

A mammal with a fishlike circulatory system would have to expend disproportionate amounts of energy to pump blood fast enough to supply its high metabolic requirements, and might therefore be regarded as inefficient compared to other mammals, but a fish equipped with a mammalian heart would have a pump far stronger than required for the work to be done. If the pump worked at anything near normal capacity, it would be supplying more oxygen than the tissues of the fish require, and this is a form of inefficiency seldom found in nature. What we customarily find is (in the words of John Hunter*) that "Nature keeps a circulation sufficient for the part, and no more."

An interesting discussion of circulatory efficiency and its relation to anatomical form is given in chapter 4 (*The Forms of Tissues*) of D'Arcy Wentworth Thompson's *On Growth and Form*.

---

*John Hunter (1728–1793) was a London surgeon who founded the first great museum of comparative anatomy. Readers interested in the history of biology will want to read his biography, *The Reluctant Surgeon*, by John Kobler (Garden City, N.Y.: Doubleday & Co., 1960).

THE RESPIRATORY SYSTEM

A considerable amount of lung tissue will have to be destroyed in the removal of the vessels directly connected with the heart, and the instructor should, therefore, direct certain students to make demonstration dissections of the lungs, leaving them intact and cutting the associated vessels as illustrated on the opposite page.

Refer to the sagittal section of the head and neck on page 21 and review the functions of the secondary palate and the epiglottis.

Examine the *trachea* and observe that it is composed of a fibrous membrane stiffened by cartilaginous rings which serve to keep the air passage open. The dorsal side of the trachea is in contact with the esophagus; in this area the cartilaginous rings are deficient, and the tube is completed by fibrous tissue and smooth muscle fibers. Each *main bronchus* divides into successively smaller branches which finally terminate in *alveoli*, minute air sacs which are richly supplied with capillaries. Exchange of oxygen and carbon dioxide occurs between the air in the alveoli and the blood in the alveolar capillaries.

The thin, serous membrane lining the lungs is the *visceral pleura*. It continues onto the inner thoracic walls and the diaphragm as the *parietal pleura*. The potential space between the lung and the inner thoracic wall is the *pleural cavity*, a division of the embryonic body cavity or celom.

In mammals, inspiration and expiration are effected by alternately increasing and decreasing the total volume of the thoracic cavity. During inspiration, the muscles which move the ribs contract and the ventral ends of the ribs are lifted with the result that the volume of the thoracic cavity is increased in the dorsoventral direction. Simultaneously, the vertical dimension of the thoracic cavity is increased by the contraction of the diaphragm, which forces the abdominal viscera downward. During expiration, the diaphragm and rib muscles relax and chest volume is diminished chiefly by the natural elasticity of the lungs and the chest wall.

The heart and lungs of the frog are not separated from the abdominal viscera by a diaphragm. The mammalian respiratory mechanism is like a suction pump, whereas the respiratory mechanism of the frog is like a force pump. The frog forces air into its lungs by closing the mouth and nares and forcibly raising the floor of the mouth. Expiration is effected by the elasticity of the lungs and by contraction of the abdominal walls.

The exchange of respiratory gases can occur across any thin, moist membrane which is exposed to the air and well supplied with capillaries. In mammals, the only surface which fulfills these requirements for respiratory exchange is the alveolar surface of the lung. In frogs, however, respiratory exchange occurs at three different sites: the skin (*cutaneous respiration*), the lungs (*pulmonary respiration*), and the mucous membrane of the mouth and pharynx (*buccopharyngeal respiration*). Pulmonary and cutaneous respiration are of comparable importance in most frogs. Cutaneous respiration accounts for somewhat more than half of the respiratory exchange in species which are chiefly aquatic; pulmonary respiration is of greater significance in frogs which spend most of their time on land. The regular oscillatory movements of the floor of the mouth are connected with olfaction as well as with buccopharyngeal respiration. Buccopharyngeal respiration does not account for a significant proportion of the respiratory exchange in most frogs, but it was undoubtedly the rule among ancient amphibians, as it still is among lungless salamanders and a few fishes which supplement gill breathing by gulping air.

Because the frog uses its mouth as a force pump, it cannot breathe while feeding, nor can it breathe if the mouth is open. This is not a disadvantage, because its low metabolism enables the frog to survive for many hours by means of cutaneous respiration alone. For a mammal, however, such a limitation would be disastrous. The movable ribs, diaphragm, epiglottis, and secondary palate are structural adaptations which make possible the constant breathing associated with the high rate of oxygen consumption and intrinsic temperature control of mammals.

Another important structural adaptation associated with intrinsic temperature control is the tremendous proliferation of the internal surface in the mammalian lung. The frog's lung is a simple sac with rudimentary internal septa. The mammalian lung, in contrast, consists of densely packed alveoli which serve to maximize the respiratory surface. In the frog, the total area across which respiratory exchange occurs is approximately one-and-a-half times the total body surface; in man, the total area of the lungs is roughly sixty-five times the body surface. A difference of the same order is found when we compare the oxygen consumption of a frog with that of a mammal of comparable weight. During maximum activity, a small mammal consumes roughly fifty times as much oxygen per gram as a frog.

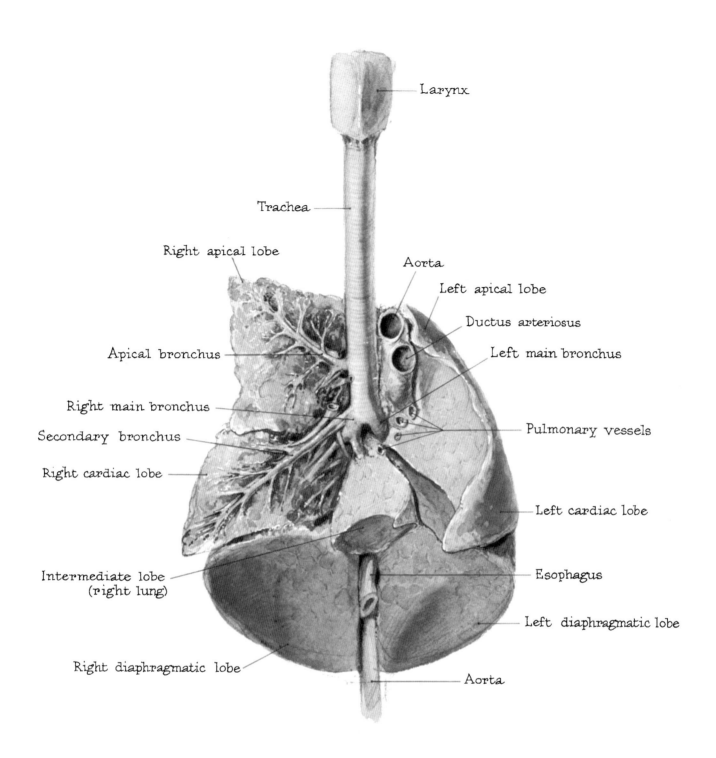

Larynx

Trachea

Right apical lobe

Aorta

Left apical lobe

Ductus arteriosus

Apical bronchus

Left main bronchus

Right main bronchus

Secondary bronchus

Pulmonary vessels

Right cardiac lobe

Left cardiac lobe

Intermediate lobe
(right lung)

Esophagus

Left diaphragmatic lobe

Right diaphragmatic lobe

Aorta

THE LUNGS, VENTRAL VIEW

The lungs are removed and the right lung is partially
dissected to show some of the branches of the right
bronchus.

THE NERVOUS SYSTEM

The brain and spinal cord are enveloped by three membranes collectively termed the *meninges*. The *dura mater* is the outermost membrane; it is tough, white, and fibrous. The *arachnoid*, or middle membrane, is delicate and weblike. It extends between the dura and the *pia mater*, or innermost membrane. The pia mater consists of a network of blood vessels and connective tissue which adheres closely to the surface of the brain and spinal cord.

To see the meninges, remove the skin from the top of the head and expose the skull. Insert the point of a stout pair of scissors in the midline and make a cut about two inches long in the sagittal plane, cutting through the skull but being careful to keep the cut shallow and not to damage the brain. Use stout forceps and scissors to remove the top of the skull on either side of the cut, exposing the dura mater, which will be seen as a sheet of white fibrous tissue between the brain and the skull. Remove the dura and expose the surface of the brain. The pia mater is the thin, transparent membrane which lies on the surface of the brain. Gently lift it with forceps and observe that it extends into the grooves (*sulci*) between the ridges (*gyri*) of the cerebral cortex. The arachnoid, which lies between the dura and the pia mater, is not easily identified on the fetal pig.

Because of its immature condition, the brain of the fetal pig is not suitable for detailed study, and the sheep brain will be used instead.

For purposes of description the brain is usually divided into three main regions: the *forebrain*, *midbrain*, and *hindbrain*. It is assumed that these regions correspond to the olfactory, optic, and auditory centers of the most primitive vertebrate ancestors, and that the functions of each region have been modified in the course of evolution.

The forebrain (primitive olfactory region) includes the *cerebrum* and the *diencephalon*. The cerebrum, which constitutes the largest part of the brain, is the center of association, memory, consciousness, and volition. Certain functions of the cerebral cortex are localized in specific areas; somatic motor and sensory areas and centers for vision,

smell, and hearing have been identified by experimental stimulation of the cerebral cortex. The convoluted surface of the cerebrum is a structural adaptation connected with the large number of association centers in the cerebral cortex. These centers facilitate the accumulation and utilization of experience, faculties which are more highly developed in mammals than in other vertebrates. Each lateral half of the cerebrum is termed a *cerebral hemisphere*. The two cerebral hemispheres are connected by a prominent commissure termed the *corpus callosum*.

The diencephalon is the region of the forebrain surrounding the third ventricle; it relays motor and sensory impulses between the cerebrum and the cranial nerves and spinal cord. It also contains optic and auditory centers, and association centers for the coordination of general visceral motor functions.

Below the diencephalon lies the hypophysis, one of the most important endocrine glands in the body. It produces hormones which control the activities of other endocrine glands and also act directly on a variety of body tissues. Among the functions controlled directly or indirectly by the hypophysis are growth, metabolism, blood pressure, and sexual development and activity.

On the dorsal surface of the diencephalon, lying just below the posterior end of the corpus callosum, is the pineal body. It represents the rudiment of the median third eye found in lampreys and certain other primitive vertebrates.

The midbrain (primitive optic region) functions in connection with the relay of motor and sensory impulses. The roof of the midbrain is expanded to form four lobes, the *corpora quadrigemina*, which mediate certain optic and auditory reflexes. The floor of the midbrain is an important center for the relay of motor impulses.

The hindbrain (primitive auditory region) consists of the *cerebellum*, *pons*, and *medulla*. The cerebellum controls muscular coordination and proprioceptive adjustment. It stores information relating to the position of the body and to sensation of equilibrium originating in the inner ear. This information is correlated with conscious motor impulses originating in the cerebral cortex to produce coordinated muscular activity.

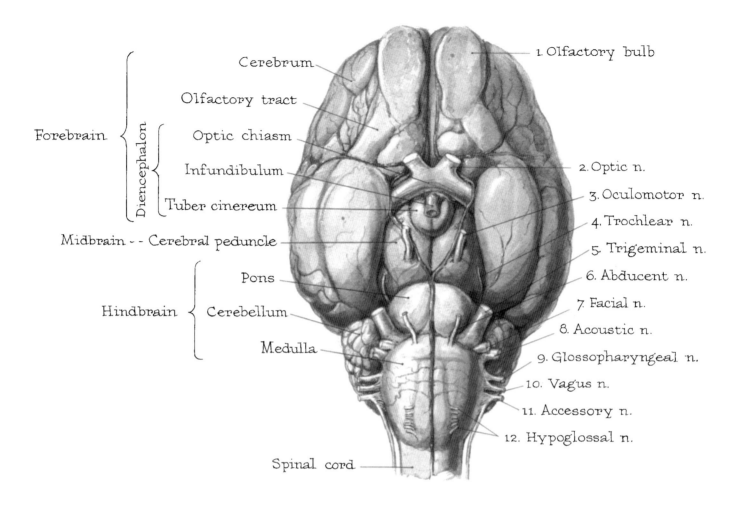

Forebrain {
    Cerebrum
    Olfactory tract
    Diencephalon {
        Optic chiasm
        Infundibulum
        Tuber cinereum
}

Midbrain - - Cerebral peduncle

Hindbrain {
    Pons
    Cerebellum
    Medulla
}

Spinal cord

1. Olfactory bulb
2. Optic n.
3. Oculomotor n.
4. Trochlear n.
5. Trigeminal n.
6. Abducent n.
7. Facial n.
8. Acoustic n.
9. Glossopharyngeal n.
10. Vagus n.
11. Accessory n.
12. Hypoglossal n.

THE SHEEP BRAIN, VENTRAL VIEW

Table of cranial nerves.

1. Olfactory. Sensory. From olfactory epithelium of nasal cavity.

2. Optic. Sensory. From eye.

3. Oculomotor. Motor. To eye muscles (superior, medial, and inferior rectus muscles and inferior oblique muscle).

4. Trochlear. Motor. To eye muscle (superior oblique).

5. Trigeminal. Sensory from head, teeth, and tongue; motor to jaw muscles.

6. Abducent. Motor. To eye muscles (lateral rectus and retractor bulbi).

7. Facial. Motor to face and neck muscles; sensory from taste buds.

8. Acoustic. Sensory. From inner ear.

9. Glossopharyngeal. Sensory and motor to tongue and pharynx.

10. Vagus. Sensory and motor to thoracic and abdominal viscera.

11. Accessory. Motor. To neck muscles.

12. Hypoglossal. Motor. Tongue and throat muscles.

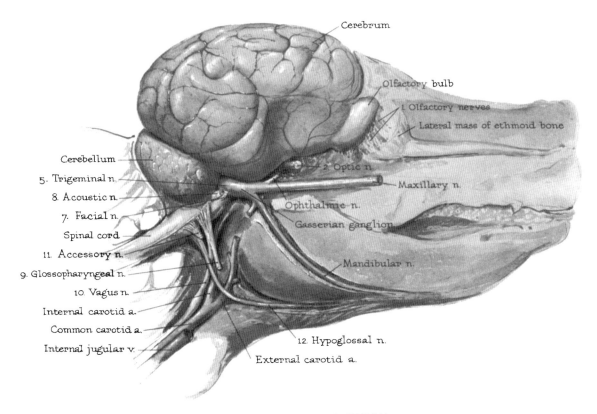

Cerebrum

Olfactory bulb

1. Olfactory nerves

Lateral mass of ethmoid bone

2. Optic n.

Maxillary n.

Ophthalmic n.

Gasserian ganglion

Mandibular n.

Cerebellum

5. Trigeminal n.

8. Acoustic n.

7. Facial n.

Spinal cord

11. Accessory n.

9. Glossopharyngeal n.

10. Vagus n.

Internal carotid a.

Common carotid a.

Internal jugular v.

12. Hypoglossal n.

External carotid a.

LATERAL VIEW OF THE BRAIN AND CRANIAL
NERVES IN THE FETAL PIG

The pons consists of fibers which connect the cerebrum, cerebellum, and medulla.

Most of the cranial nerves originate from the medulla. Within it are centers controlling involuntary functions such as heartbeat, respiration, vasoconstriction, and swallowing.

Refer to page 60 and attempt to identify the cranial nerves on your specimen. The nerves are delicate and easily torn during the removal of the brain; you may therefore be unable to find some of the roots.

The cranial nerves may be gouped in three categories: special sensory nerves, which are purely sensory; branchial nerves, which for the most part carry both sensory and motor impulses; and somatic motor nerves, which are purely motor.

Nerves 1, 2, and 8 are termed *special sensory nerves*; they carry impulses which are subjectively perceived as sensations of smell, sight, and sound, respectively. In primitive vertebrates, a pair of sensory nerves presumably originated from each of the three main regions of the brain: olfactory nerves from the forebrain, optic nerves from the midbrain, and acoustic nerves from the hindbrain. A reflection of this pattern may be seen in the mammalian brain. The olfactory nerves enter the cerebrum, or most anterior part of the forebrain. The optic nerves enter the diencephalon, very close to the midbrain, and their impulses go to primary visual centers in the midbrain and diencephalon. From these centers, the impulses are relayed to the cerebrum, the site of conscious visual sensation in mammals. The acoustic nerve goes to the hindbrain, and impulses from the inner ear are relayed to the cerebrum, site of conscious perception of sound, and to the cerebellum, coordinating center for the maintenance of normal equilibrium.

The somatic motor nerves include nerves 3, 4, and 6, which innervate the eye muscles, and nerve 12, which innervates the muscles of the tongue. These nerves are comparable in many respects to the ventral, or motor, roots of spinal nerves (note the ventral origin of the roots of nerve 12).

Nerves 5, 7, 9, 10, and 11 are termed branchial nerves. Observe that all the branchial nerves originate from the medulla and that, except for 10, they are largely concerned with the innervation of the head and neck muscles. The branchial nerves have evolved from spinal nerves

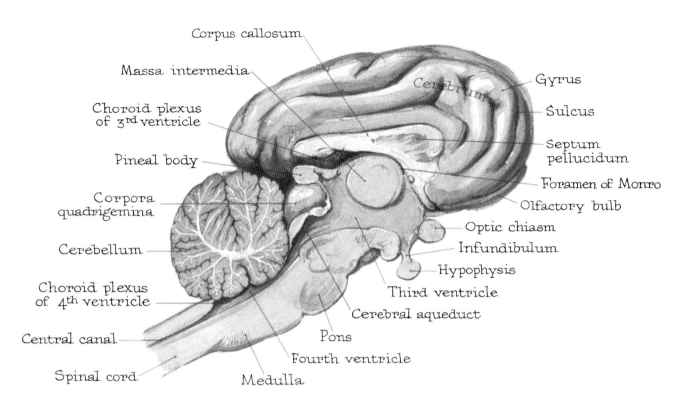

Corpus callosum

Massa intermedia

Choroid plexus
of 3rd ventricle

Pineal body

Corpora
quadrigemina

Cerebellum

Choroid plexus
of 4th ventricle

Central canal

Spinal cord

Cerebrum

Gyrus

Sulcus

Septum
pellucidum

Foramen of Monro

Olfactory bulb

Optic chiasm

Infundibulum

Hypophysis

Third ventricle

Cerebral aqueduct

Pons

Fourth ventricle

Medulla

SAGITTAL SECTION OF THE SHEEP BRAIN

which innervated the gill and neck muscles of primitive vertebrates. The primitive branchial nerve pattern has been greatly modified with the evolution of the jaw and neck muscles as seen in mammals. The anterior portion of the spinal cord from which these nerves originated in primitive vertebrates has been incorporated into the hindbrain, and the nerves have migrated toward the brain. The crowding of the branchial nerves at the anterior end of the medulla is often cited as an example of the fact that the cell bodies of neurons tend to migrate toward the source of strongest stimulation, a phenomenon termed *neurobiotaxis*.

After identifying the cranial nerves, cut the brain in the sagittal plane and identify the structures illustrated above.

The brain and spinal cord originate embryonically as a hollow tube, and the cavity of the primitive neural tube develops into the ventricles of the brain and the central canal of the spinal cord. The two cerebral hemispheres contain cavities termed the *first* and *second*, or *lateral*, *ventricles*. Each lateral ventricle communicates with the median *third ventricle* by an opening termed the *foramen of Monro*. Probe the foramen of Monro and trim away the septum pellucidum to see one of the lateral ventricles.

Within the lateral ventricle you will find a delicate vascular membrane, the *choroid plexus of the lateral ventricle*. Choroid plexuses will also be found in the third and fourth ventricles. The choroid plexuses represent a fusion of the pia mater with the inner epithelial lining of the central canal and ventricles. Exchange of nutrient substances and other materials takes place between the choroid plexuses and the slowly circulating, lymphlike cerebrospinal fluid. This fluid fills the ventricles and the central canal of the spinal cord as well as the space between the dura mater and the brain and spinal cord.

It is possible to demonstrate the spinal cord and the spinal nerves in the fetal pig, but because of the small size of the structures involved and the difficulty of removing the surrounding muscle and bone, this portion of the nervous system may best be studied by reference to a demonstration dissection, models, and illustrations.

The *spinal cord* lies within the vertebral canal. It is a tubular structure containing a small *central canal* which extends throughout its length. Anteriorly, the central canal is continuous with the fourth ventricle of the brain and posteriorly it ends in the *filum terminale*, or slender distal end of the spinal cord.

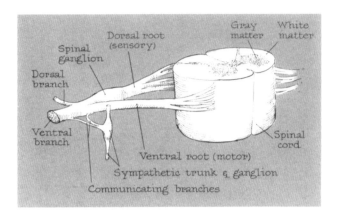

In cross section, the spinal cord is seen to consist of two types of material, *gray matter* and *white matter*. Gray matter consists largely of the cell bodies of neurons. It is within the gray matter that associative and reflex functions occur. White matter, which forms the external portion of the spinal cord, consists of message-carrying fibers. Its whitish appearance is due to the fact that these fibers are surrounded by sheaths of fatty, nonconductive material termed *myelin*, which serves to insulate the nerve fibers much as rubber insulates an electric wire. In the cerebrum, cerebellum, and certain other areas of the brain, the relative positions of gray and white matter are reversed, so that the gray matter is peripheral to the white matter.

Each *spinal nerve* arises from the spinal cord by a dorsal and a ventral root. The dorsal root carries sensory impulses only, and is supplied with a ganglion which contains the cell bodies of the sensory neurons. The ventral root carries motor impulses only and has no ganglion. The cell bodies of the motor neurons lie within the gray matter of the spinal cord. The dorsal and ventral roots unite to form the spinal nerve, which emerges through the intervertebral foramen and divides into three branches: a small *dorsal branch*, which supplies the muscles and skin of the dorsal part of the body; a large *ventral branch*, which supplies the muscles and skin of the ventral and lateral parts of the body, including the limbs, and one or more small *communicating* branches, which join ganglia of the autonomic system and supply the viscera.

There are thirty-three spinal nerves in the pig, named according to the regions of the vertebral column through which they exit: eight *cervical*, fourteen *thoracic*, seven *lumbar*, and four *sacral*. The number of spinal nerves varies somewhat among different vertebrates. In man there are thirty-one; in the horse, forty-two.

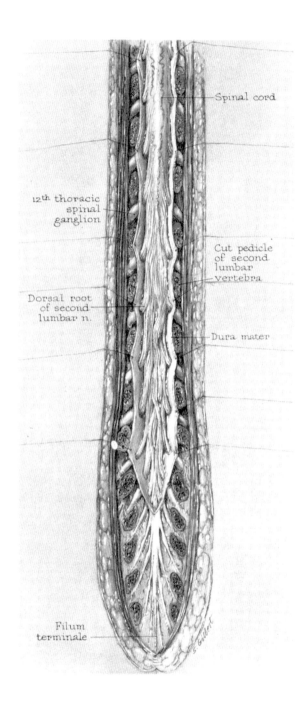

THE HUMAN CAUDA EQUINA

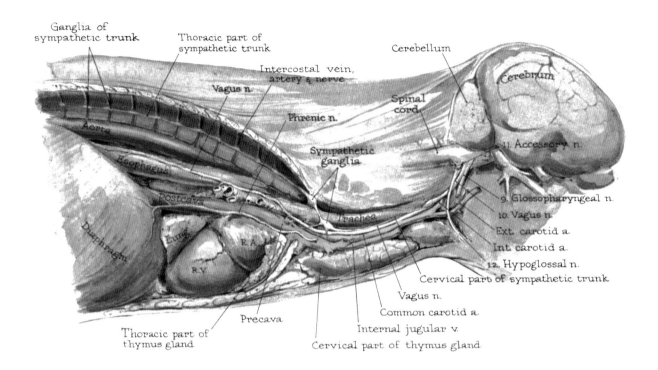

Ganglia of
sympathetic trunk

Thoracic part of
sympathetic trunk

Intercostal vein,
artery & nerve

Vagus n.

Phrenic n.

Cerebellum

Cerebrum

Spinal
cord

Aorta

Esophagus

Postcava

Sympathetic
ganglia

11. Accessory n.

9. Glossopharyngeal n.

10. Vagus n.

Ext. carotid a.

Int. carotid a.

Trachea

12. Hypoglossal n.

Diaphragm

Lung

R.A.

R.V.

Cervical part of sympathetic trunk

Vagus n.

Common carotid a.

Internal jugular v.

Cervical part of thymus gland

Precava

Thoracic part of
thymus gland

THE PHRENIC AND VAGUS NERVES

The phrenic nerve (motor nerve to the diaphragm) originates
from the ventral branches of the sixth and seventh cervical nerves.

The roots of each spinal nerve originate somewhat anterior to the intervertebral foramen through which the nerve exits. The roots of the anterior nerves lie close to the foramina through which they exit, but the roots of the posterior nerves lie relatively farther away, with the result that in the lower part of the vertebral canal, the roots of the nerves lie parallel to each other and may extend for some distance within the canal before making their exits. The spinal cord does not extend to the end of the vertebral canal; in the pig it extends to the sacrum, but in man it extends only to the first or second lumbar vertebra. The roots of the lower spinal nerves extend beyond the end of the spinal cord and are collectively termed the *cauda equina*.

Both the sizes of the spinal nerves and of the spinal cord vary in proportion to the amount of tissue innervated. In all tetrapods, the spinal cord exhibits two distinct swellings: the cervical enlargement, which corresponds to the attachments of the large nerves which supply the forelimbs, and the lumbar enlargement, corresponding to the attachments of the nerves which supply the hindlimbs. The nerves supplying the limbs form complex networks, or *plexuses*, after leaving the vertebral canal. The network

of nerves supplying the forelimb is termed the *brachial plexus*; that supplying the hindlimbs is termed the *lumbo-sacral plexus*.

The innervation of the viscera is effected by the *autonomic nervous system*, which carries involuntary motor impulses exclusively. The autonomic system consists of two subdivisions which have mutually antagonistic effects: the *sympathetic* and the *parasympathetic systems*. Impulses mediated by the sympathetic system are associated with emergency reactions such as fear and flight. Examples of its effects are dilation of the pupils, increased heart rate and blood pressure, slowing of peristalsis, and dilation of the bronchioles. Impulses mediated by the parasympathetic system reverse each of the above effects and restore the organism to the resting state.

Parasympathetic innervation of the thoracic and abdominal viscera is effected by fibers associated with the vagus nerve and by fibers which emerge by way of the spinal nerves in the pelvic region. (See the course of the vagus nerve as illustrated above; also see a demonstration dissection made by your instructor.)

That portion of the sympathetic system which can be easily identified in the fetal pig consists of the sympathetic trunks, thin strands of nerve tissue lying on either side of the vertebral column and extending from the base of the skull to the coccyx. Each sympathetic trunk is connected with the spinal nerves and the spinal cord by small communicating branches. Branches also extend from the sympathetic trunk to the thoracic and abdominal viscera, and these branches commonly pass through autonomic nerve plexuses before reaching their destinations. One such plexus is the celiac plexus; you noticed this as a mass of tough white tissue surrounding the celiac and anterior mesenteric arteries during your dissection of the abdominal vessels. Most of the branches and plexuses of the autonomic system are too small to be identified in the fetal pig, and this part of the nervous system may best be studied by reference to diagrams in general texts.

In comparing the brain of the sheep with that of the frog, we find the most striking difference in the tremendous size of the mammalian cerebrum and cerebellum. The optic lobes, which constitute a prominent part of the frog's brain, are homologous with the relatively insignificant anterior lobes of the corpora quadrigemina in the sheep's brain. The relatively large size of the cerebrum and cerebellum in mammals is a structural adaptation connected with the tremendous increase of association centers in the cerebral cortex and with the capacity for varied responses, learning, and complex coordinated muscular reactions.

The importance of the mammalian cerebrum is indicated by the fact that if it is surgically removed in an experimental animal, the animal is reduced to a vegetative state. In contrast, frogs in which the forebrain has been removed exhibit a certain lack of spontaneity, but are able to feed, swim, and breed much as normal frogs do.

In frogs, the optic lobes control complex behavior and are the regions of highest integration. Most terminal fibers of the frog's visual system are received by the optic lobes, whereas in mammals visual impulses are relayed to the posterior part of the cerebral cortex, which is the site of conscious visual perception. Electrical stimulation of the optic lobes of the frog elicits movements of the body and limbs; in mammals such movements are elicited by stimulation of certain localized areas of the cerebral cortex. Stimulation of the frog's cerebrum produces no movements of the body or limbs.

Although it is sometimes implied that motor responses originate in the frog's optic lobes and that these lobes are the centers of vision and of consciousness, it is interesting to find that considerable portions of the optic lobes may be removed without apparent impairment of vision, and that frogs in which this operation has been performed are capable of many of the actions normally associated with conscious volition. Holmes reports that "removal of the optic lobes was found to produce forced movements, an abnormal retention of urine, and a slight loss of sight, but later these symptoms gradually disappeared," and he adds that frogs in which this operation has been performed are still capable of coordinated jumping and swimming movements. Even if the cerebellum and all portions of the brain anterior to it are removed, the frog is still capable of coordinated locomotion, the snapping reflex, and a number of other reactions.

Such experiments illustrate the point that in lower vertebrates the spinal cord is capable of initiating a number of autonomous responses. This capacity is much diminished in higher vertebrates. In fish, the spinal cord is the site of complex chain reflexes and is capable of transmitting coordinated wave patterns independently of the brain. If the spinal cord of a dogfish shark is cut behind the brain, the shark is still able to swim in an essentially normal manner. If the spinal cord of a cat is cut in the upper thoracic region, the cat is unable to walk or stand. As the brain increases in importance, the capacity of the spinal cord to initiate independent responses diminishes. The evolution of forebrain dominance as seen in mammals is a reflection of a general evolutionary trend toward cephalization and specialization of function.

If the brains of the frog and the sheep are cut in cross section, it will be seen that in the cerebrum of the frog the gray matter is internal and the white matter is external, the same condition found in the spinal cord. In the mammalian cerebrum, these relations are reversed; the gray matter (cerebral cortex) is external and the white matter is internal. Gray matter is external to white matter in all vertebrate cerebellums. The externalization of the cerebral gray matter is a progressive trend originating in reptiles and culminating in mammals.

This trend may be interpreted in terms of the metabolic requirements of the brain, which are substantial compared with those of many other body tissues. In a normal young human adult, the brain accounts for about 20 per cent of the total basal body oxygen consumption, although it represents only about 2 per cent of the total body weight. Even higher rates are found in children. In a five-year-old, the brain, which has already reached near-adult proportions, may require as much as half the total oxygen consumed by the body at rest.

The rate of oxygen consumption varies within different parts of the brain itself. Gray matter, which consists chiefly of cell bodies of neurons, is metabolically more active than white matter and therefore requires a more efficient blood supply. Studies of the living cat brain show that blood flow to the gray matter is about five times greater than blood flow to the white matter. The tissue of the brain is exceptionally dense, and its blood supply comes exclusively from vessels of superficial origin. The interstitial space (which in other tissues contains the extracellular fluid, or internal environment) is minimal in brain tissue. The peripheral position and the convoluted surface of the cerebral cortex in mammals therefore serve two important functions: They put that part of the brain which needs the most oxygen into close contact with the superficial blood vessels, and at the same time expose it to the cerebrospinal fluid, which constitutes the internal environment of the brain.

The oxygen requirements of the brain are also reflected in the circulatory system. A review of the circulatory mechanisms of the fish, frog, and mammal reveals that in each case the brain is supplied with the most highly oxygenated blood available. In the case of the fetal circulation, this mechanism is particularly significant; almost all the most highly oxygenated blood goes first to the brain, then back to the heart again before being sent to the body.

In connection with the form and the metabolic requirements of the brain, it is interesting to find that there is a fundamental relationship between absolute brain size and total metabolism, and that this relationship embraces both warm-blooded and cold-blooded forms, including many invertebrates (but excluding man and the higher primates). The relationship may be expressed as the ratio between the brain weight in grams and the total calorie production during twenty-four hours. In a wide range of animals, this ratio averages 1 to 12.115. This means that most animals, when resting, produce about twelve calories per day for every gram of brain weight. The brain of a five-pound rabbit, for instance, is comparable in weight to the brain of a 240-pound alligator. In both animals the brain weighs about eight grams, and in both animals heat production is about one hundred calories per day. Some of the implications of this interesting relationship, together with a discussion of the connection between metabolism, form, and habitat are given by George Crile in his book *Intelligence, Power and Personality* (McGraw-Hill, 1941).

We have seen that in many cases it is possible to relate structural differences between the frog and the pig to the fact that the frog is a cold-blooded vertebrate and the pig is a warm-blooded vertebrate. Is it also possible to relate the development of intelligent behavior to the warm-blooded mode of life? Are there any physical factors which favor the evolution of intelligence in warm-blooded, rather than in cold-blooded, animals?

One such factor is the speed of the nerve impulse. Nerve impulses travel faster at high temperatures than they do at low temperatures. In most cases the speed of the impulse doubles for each rise in temperature of 10°C. The speed of the impulse is also influenced by the size of the nerve fiber. A fiber of fifteen or twenty microns in diameter may conduct up to one hundred times faster than a fiber one micron in diameter. Thus both the size of the fibers and the temperatures at which they operate may have played a role in the evolution of intelligence in warm-blooded forms.

It is a commonplace observation that in warm-blooded animals the brain constitutes a relatively greater proportion of the body weight than it does in cold-blooded animals, and Crile's tabulation of brain weight and metabolism shows that there is a fairly high degree of correlation between absolute brain size and total heat production. It is also a basic observation that the size of nervous system components varies with the degree of activity of the structures innervated. Many examples of this may be found. The spinal cord of a fish is uniform throughout in diameter, but the spinal cords of tetrapods exhibit swellings at the points where the spinal nerves innervating the forelimbs and hindlimbs attach to the cord. In certain blind, burrowing amphibians, the sense of smell is dominant; in these animals, the forebrain is large and the optic lobes are small. In the eye-minded frog, the reverse is normally true, but if the eyes of a tadpole are destroyed the optic lobes do not develop to normal size. The size of the cerebellum is considerable in animals which perform complex coordinated movements, but small in animals which are capable only of relatively stereotyped muscular responses. These and similar observations suggest that the high metabolic rate and sustained physical activity of primitive mammals were conditions which favored the evolution of large brains and intelligent behavior.

In this connection it is interesting to find that the earliest mammals were on the whole no more intelligent than their reptilian contemporaries. A characteristically mammalian level of intelligence evolved *after* the evolution of intrinsic temperature control, and it evolved independently in various mammalian groups.

Before we allow ourselves to become inordinately proud of our high temperatures and our ten-billion-neuron brains, however, it may be well to make the sobering observation that the ant exhibits marvelously organized social and economic behavior which includes such characteristically human activities as farming, keeping domestic animals, making war, and taking slaves. It happens that in mammals large brains, intrinsic temperature control, and intelligence have evolved together and are functionally related. Birds, however, have become warm-blooded without becoming remarkably intelligent, and there is no doubt that various forms of intelligence might evolve under conditions entirely different from those in which mammals have lived for the last seventy million years. The form of intelligence which has evolved in humans is the direct development of patterns of social action which had survival value for early primates in the bio-physical environment peculiar to them, and our view of the world is conditioned, enriched, and limited by this heritage.

An excellent descriptive survey covering past and recent work on the physiology of the brain is given in Dean E. Wooldridge's *The Machinery of the Brain* (McGraw-Hill paperback, 1963).

THE EYE

Make a horizontal cut around the circumference of the beef eye. Do not attempt to cut the lens. Place the eye in a dish of water and examine it, identifying the structures illustrated on the opposite page.

The eyeball is usually described as consisting of three concentric tunics or layers. The *external tunic* is composed of the *sclera* and the *cornea*. The sclera is the "white" of the eye. It is an opaque protective covering composed of white fibrous tissue intermixed with elastic fibers. The sclera is continuous in front with the transparent cornea, through which light enters the eye.

The *vascular middle tunic* is composed of the *iris*, *ciliary body*, and *choroid*. The choroid is a pigmented and richly vascular layer which carries nutriment for the highly metabolic retina. The ciliary body consists of a thickened portion of the vascular tunic plus the ciliary muscle, a circular band of involuntary muscle fibers which function in accommodation. The pigmented iris, which is continuous with the choroid and the ciliary body, represents a fusion of the anterior part of the vascular tunic and the anterior, nonsensory portion of the retina. It contains involuntary muscle fibers which respond to autonomic nervous control and regulate the amount of light which falls on the retina by modifying the size of the pupil.

The *retina* is the photoreceptive inner tunic of the eye. The sensory layer of the retina contains two types of cells: rods and cones. Rods function in the perception of faint light and give poorly defined black-and-white images. Cones function under conditions of good illumination, give good visual details, and, in some animals, respond to color. Man and the higher primates have good color vision; in most other mammals color vision is minimal or absent. The area of most acute vision is the *area centralis*, which lies in the posterior part of the retina in line with the optical axis of the eye. Cones are most numerous in the area centralis, whereas rods predominate in the periphery of the retina.

The cavities of the eye contain fluids termed the *aqueous humor* (anterior to the lens) and the *vitreous humor* (posterior to the lens). These fluids maintain a constant pressure which keeps the external tunic of the eye distended to the point of rigidity. The aqueous humor, which is more fluid than the vitreous humor, is constantly secreted at a slow rate by the epithelium of the ciliary body and is drained out of the eyeball into the bloodstream in such a way as to regulate the intraocular pressure and maintain the turgidity of the eyeball.

Some mammals are capable of changing the curvature, and thus the focus, of the lens. This process is termed *accommodation* and is best developed in man. Other mammals capable of accommodation are the higher apes, baboons, cats, and semiaquatic and aquatic mammals such as the whale, seal, and otter.

In mammals, accommodation is effected by contraction of the ciliary muscle. When the ciliary muscle is relaxed, the tension resulting from the normal turgidity of the eye is transmitted to the lens via the suspensory ligament, which attaches the lens to the ciliary body. This tension results in a flattening of the lens. When the ciliary muscle contracts, the tension is released and the lens, by virtue of its natural elasticity, assumes a more curved shape. This shortens the focal length of the lens and brings images of nearby objects into focus.

Movements of the eye are effected by seven muscles. There are four bandlike rectus muscles which arise around the optic foramen (the opening through which the optic nerve enters the orbit), diverge to embrace the eyeball, and insert on the sclera. The *rectus muscles* are named according to their positions relative to the eyeball (*superior*, *inferior*, *medial*, and *lateral*). Two *oblique muscles* (*superior* and *inferior*) originate from the anterior part of the orbit and insert respectively on the superior and inferior parts of the eyeball. In addition, there is a *retractor bulbi muscle* which retracts the eyeball (this muscle is absent in primates).

Pull the retina away from the choroid and observe the *tapetum lucidum*, a semicircular area of bright, lustrous tissue which occupies a considerable portion of the choroid above the optic nerve. The tapetum is an adaptation for vision in limited light. The familiar eyeshine seen when car lights are reflected in the eyes of a cat at night is

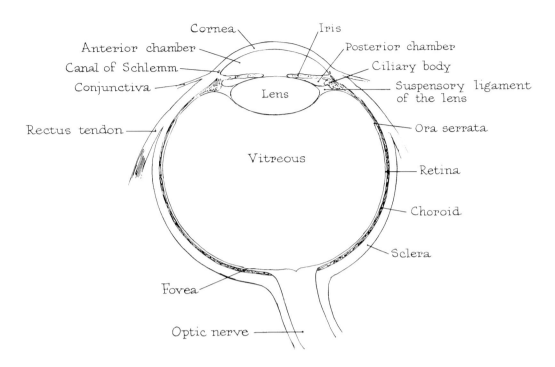

Cornea

Iris

Anterior chamber

Posterior chamber

Canal of Schlemm

Ciliary body

Conjunctiva

Suspensory ligament
of the lens

Lens

Rectus tendon

Ora serrata

Vitreous

Retina

Choroid

Sclera

Fovea

Optic nerve

HUMAN EYE, HORIZONTAL SECTION

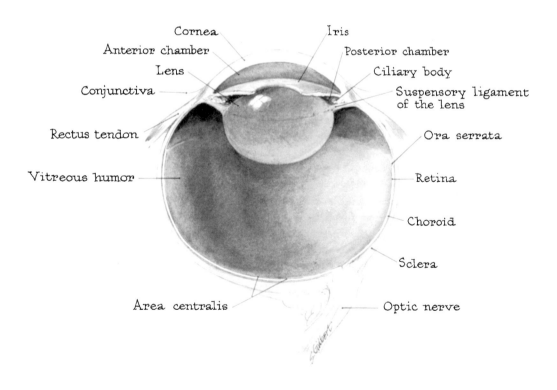

Cornea

Iris

Anterior chamber

Posterior chamber

Lens

Ciliary body

Conjunctiva

Suspensory ligament
of the lens

Rectus tendon

Ora serrata

Vitreous humor

Retina

Choroid

Sclera

Area centralis

Optic nerve

BEEF EYE, HORIZONTAL SECTION

due to the presence of the tapetum, which is found in many nocturnal animals. In the eye which lacks a tapetum, light passes through the retina and is absorbed by the pigmented choroid. In the eye which has a tapetum, light passes through the retina twice, once coming in and once again when it is reflected back. Thus apparent contrast is enhanced and night vision is facilitated. A variety of tapeta have evolved, been lost, and evolved again in the course of evolution. Tapeta are found in some sharks, teleosts, reptiles, and marsupials, as well as in many mammals, and eyeshine of undetermined origin is reported in many animals which lack a true tapetum.

It is possible to construct a camera in which the principle of the tapetum is used to make photographs in dim light. In such a camera, the emulsion is on the back of the plate and is in contact with a mirror which reflects the image back through the emulsion. Such cameras are not in general use; when a photographer wants to take a picture at night he customarily uses artificial light or takes a time exposure. In the eye, a time exposure cannot be made to serve instead of good illumination, and therefore the tapetum is the customary adaptation among animals requiring good vision at night.

The value of the tapetum to the cat, which often hunts at night, seems obvious, but what purpose does the tapetum serve in ungulates (hoofed herbivores)? The answer to this question has to do with the fact that ungulates are the prey of large carnivores. The ungulate doesn't need the tapetum to see its food, but to see its enemies. It is essential for the defenseless ungulate to be able to see and recognize an enemy at the greatest possible distance. Even if the light is moderately good, the retinal image of a distant object is dimmer than that of a nearby object. The tapetum, therefore, probably facilitates distance vision as well as night vision.

The beef eye exhibits other structural adaptations which are related to the predator-prey relationship between ungulates and carnivores. Examine a beef eye in which the cornea and lens are intact and observe the horizontally oblong shape of the pupil. This shape extends the field of vision afforded by the lateral orientation of the eyes, increasing the extent of the binocular field to the front and also the range of peripheral vision to the rear. Compare the pupil of the beef eye with that of the cat's eye.

The lateral orientation of the eyes in ungulates affords a wide field of view and thus a good chance to see an approaching predator. Laterally oriented eyes are also found in rabbits, mice, and many other defenseless animals. The tendency toward frontal orientation of the eyes and a large binocular field is characteristic of cats, owls, and many other predators which need to have the best possible view of their prey for effective pursuit.

The eyes of ungulates which live in the wild are permanently adjusted for distance vision and have little or no ability to focus on nearby objects. This is no disadvantage, however; a grazing animal does not need to bring leaves and grass into sharp focus. While eating, however, it does need to watch the distant edge of the forest, where predators may be lurking. Most cats, on the other hand, are capable of some accommodation. Binocular vision and accommodation are adaptations which enable them to judge distance and to pursue moving prey effectively. They are agile runners, capable of great bursts of speed over short distances but incapable of sustained running over long distances. Given adequate warning, the zebra can escape the lion by running. The eyes and running habits of cats are associated with maneuverability and short bursts of great speed; the eyes and running habits of ungulates are associated with endurance and sustained running in a straight line. These adaptations are reflected in the fact that matadors fight bulls, but not lions. A man can learn to sidestep a charging bull, but would be easy prey for the binocular vision and agility of the lion.

In comparing the frog's eye with the beef eye, perhaps the first thing to be noticed is that the eye of the frog is relatively large. The ratio of eye weight to body weight in the bullfrog is 1:200; in the cow it is on the order of 1:8,000. The comparison of retinal areas shows that the retinal area of the bullfrog is about 1/10 that of the cow. Why does the bullfrog need such large eyes? Since it feeds exclusively on small prey, wouldn't smaller eyes do just as well?

One of the factors influencing the relatively large size of the eyes in frogs and many other small animals is that the diameter of the visual cells in the retina varies only within fairly narrow limits. Absolute eye size affects visual acuity because small retinas, in general, contain fewer visual cells than large retinas. The image seen by a frog is analogous to a photograph reproduced by coarse halftone dots, whereas the image seen by the cow is analogous to a photograph reproduced by fine halftone dots.

The eyes of the frog and the cow differ in proportion as well as in size. The lens of the frog eye is close to the retina, relatively large, and almost spherical. The lens of the cow's eye is farther from the retina, relatively small, and much flatter than the frog's. The frog's eye is like a camera with a wide-angle lens and a very short focal length. The broad, curved cornea, the almost spherical lens, and the potentially large pupil enable the frog's eye to take in a wide field of view, transmit a maximum amount of light, and cast a bright retinal image. These optical properties are adapted to the frog's way of life. The wide field of view and the upward orientation of the eyes enable the frog to remain motionless and see prey or predators approaching from any direction. The light-gathering power of the eye facilitates vision at night, when many frogs are most active. The spherical lens casts relatively large images of nearby objects and relatively small images of distant objects, and is capable of accommodating by moving forward to focus on insects which come within snapping distance. Frogs do not have good distance vision because the lens forms small images of distant objects and the total number of visual cells is relatively small. Any large object which comes into the frog's field of view is a sign to take cover or leap into the water.

The lens of the beef eye has a relatively long focal length and is therefore farther from the retina than the lens of the frog's eye. It takes in a narrower field of view and casts a dimmer retinal image, but it forms large and clearly focused images of distant objects and has superior resolving power because of its large absolute size.

The frog's method of accommodation is related to its method of feeding and to the structure of its lens. Because the focal length of the lens is short, a slight amount of shift in lens position is sufficient to bring the image of a nearby object into focus. The spherical shape and the small absolute size of the frog's lens make it relatively rigid. Considerable pressure would be required to change its shape, and therefore a slight change in lens-to-retina distance is apparently a method of accommodation well adapted to the structure of the frog's eye. This method is not suitable, however, for eyes with lenses of long focal length. The longer the focal length, the greater the change in lens-to-retina distance which is required to effect accommodation. If the focal length of the lens is very long, as it is in the human eye, the distance the lens would have to move to accommodate for nearby objects becomes impractically large.

The classic work on the vertebrate eye is Gordon Walls' *The Vertebrate Eye and Its Adaptive Radiation* (Hafner Publishing Co., 1963), a rich source of information which should be of interest to every student of zoology. Walls writes:

If the comparative ophthalmologists of the world should ever hold a convention, the first resolution they would pass would say: "Everything in the vertebrate eye means something." Except for the brain, there is no other organ in the body of which that can be said. It does not matter in the least whether a liver has three lobes or four, or whether the tip of the heart points north or south, or whether a hand has five fingers or six, or whether a kidney is long and narrow or short and wide. But if we should make comparable changes in the makeup of a vertebrate eye, we should quite destroy its usefulness. Man can make optical instruments only from such materials as brass and glass. Nature has succeeded with only such things as leather and water and jelly. The resulting instrument is so delicately balanced that it will tolerate no tampering.

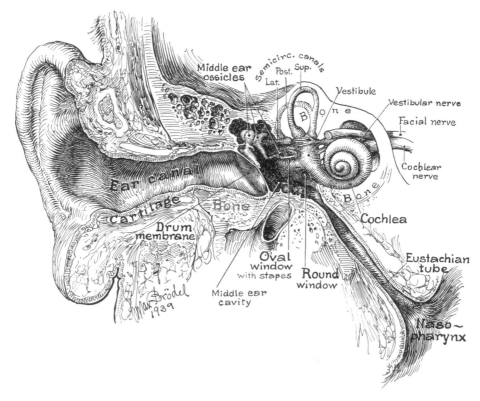

THE HUMAN EAR

This illustration by Max Broedel represents a reconstruction based on serial sections of several specimens. (Reproduced by permission of W. B. Saunders Co.)

THE EAR

The dissection of the ear in the fetal pig is complicated by the small size of the structures involved and by the fact that the inner ear is embedded in bone. The ear may, therefore, best be studied by reference to illustrations, models, and a demonstration dissection by the instructor.

The ear, or organ of hearing and equilibration, may be described as consisting of three parts: (1) *the external ear*, consisting of the pinna (cartilaginous portion outside the head) and the external auditory canal; (2) the *middle ear*, consisting of the tympanum (eardrum), the middle ear cavity within the temporal bone, and the auditory ossicles; (3) the *inner ear*, consisting of a cavity within the petrous temporal bone and a membranous labyrinth of sacs and ducts which lie within this cavity.

The *pinna* serves to direct and concentrate high-frequency sound waves by reflection. In animals such as the cat and the rabbit, movement of the pinna also aids in the localization of sound. The external auditory canal affords protection for the delicate tympanum.

The *tympanum* vibrates in response to sound waves in air, and its vibrations are conveyed to the inner ear by the *middle ear ossicles*, an articulated chain of three minute bones: the *malleus* (hammer), *incus* (anvil), and *stapes* (stirrup). The malleus is attached to the tympanum and the incus lies between the malleus and the stapes. The medial end of the stapes fits into the *oval window*, one of two openings in the temporal bone between the cavities of the middle and inner ear. The other opening is the *round window*, located near the oval window and covered by a thin membrane.

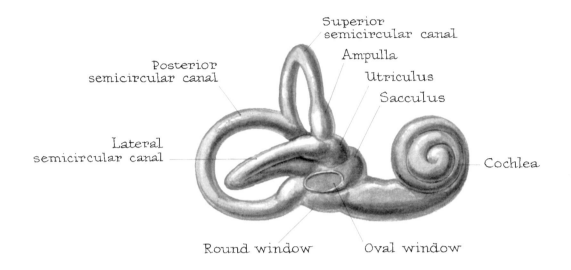

Superior
semicircular canal

Ampulla

Utriculus

Sacculus

Posterior
semicircular canal

Lateral
semicircular canal

Cochlea

Round window

Oval window

THE BONY LABYRINTH

Lateral view of a cast of the right bony labyrinth, a cavity
within the petrous temporal bone. The membranous labyrinth,
or essential organ of hearing, lies within this cavity. (After
Sobotta.)

The cavity of the inner ear is connected with the pharynx by the *Eustachian tube,* which serves to equalize pressure between the cavity of the middle ear and the surrounding air.

The inner ear consists of the *bony labyrinth,* which is a cavity within the petrous temporal bone, and the *membranous labyrinth,* which is a delicate membranous system of ducts and sacs. The membranous labyrinth lies within the bony labyrinth and closely resembles it in shape. The space between the membranous labyrinth and the bony labyrinth is filled with a clear, lymphlike fluid, the *perilymph.* The membranous labyrinth itself is filled with a similar fluid, the *endolymph.* The ramifications of the acoustic nerve (cranial nerve 8) terminate in sensory areas located in the walls of the membranous labyrinth.

Vibrations of the middle ear ossicles are conveyed to the *cochlea,* that portion of the membranous labyrinth which is specialized for the perception of sound. Pressure waves in the fluid within the cochlea stimulate receptors which initiate impulses in the acoustic nerve; these impulses are subjectively perceived as sound.

Because fluid is almost incompressible, the pressure waves in the cochlear fluid must have an escape valve. Such a valve is provided by the round window, which is connected with the oval window by way of a duct which extends throughout the entire length of the cochlea. Thus outgoing vibrations have a different pathway from incoming vibrations. The incoming vibrations are transmitted directly via the ossicles, but the outgoing vibrations are released into the air of the middle ear cavity.

The portions of the membranous labyrinth which are specialized for the perception of position and motion are the *sacculus, utriculus,* and *semicircular canals.* The sacculus and utriculus are saclike structures each of which contains a sensory patch termed a *macula.* Fine crystals of calcium carbonate (termed *otoconia*) are imbedded in a mucoid material overlying the macula. Changes in the position of the body cause changes in the force exerted by the otoconia on the sensory cells of the maculae. These changes initiate acoustic nerve impulses which are functional in equilibration.

The semicircular canals lie in mutually perpendicular planes. At one end of each canal is an ampulla containing a sensory area termed a *crista.* Each semicircular canal registers angular acceleration in the plane in which it lies.

In the frog, there is no external ear. The tympanum lies at the surface of the head, and its vibrations are conveyed to the inner ear by a single cylindrical ossicle, the *columella.* The medial end of the columella fits into an oval window, as in mammals, but there is no round window. Vibrations of the columella are conveyed to the sound-perceiving portion of the membranous labyrinth via a membranous fluid-filled canal termed the *perilymphatic*

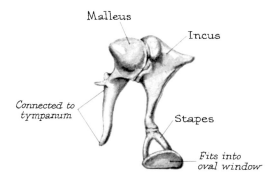

Malleus

Incus

Connected to tympanum

Stapes

Fits into oval window

THE MIDDLE EAR OSSICLES

(After a photograph in David L. Bassett's *Stereoscopic Atlas of Human Anatomy*, by permission of the author.)

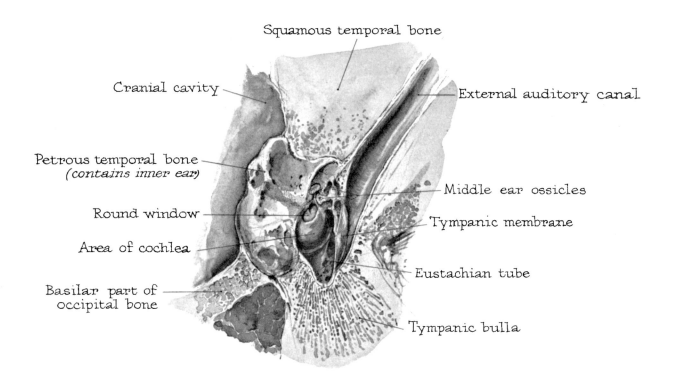

Squamous temporal bone

Cranial cavity

External auditory canal

Petrous temporal bone *(contains inner ear)*

Middle ear ossicles

Round window

Tympanic membrane

Area of cochlea

Eustachian tube

Basilar part of occipital bone

Tympanic bulla

POSTERIOR VIEW OF THE EXTERNAL AUDITORY CANAL AND THE MIDDLE EAR IN AN ADULT PIG

The temporal bone is cut away to reveal the external auditory canal and the middle ear ossicles. The dissection of the middle and inner ear is complicated by the fact that the membranous labyrinth is embedded in the petrous temporal bone and cannot be readily demonstrated in a gross specimen.

duct. The escape valve for pressure waves in the perilymphatic duct is an opening between the capsule of the inner ear and the brain.

The membranous labyrinth of the frog is similar to that of the mammal except that in the frog there is no cochlea. Sound perception occurs in one or more small sensory areas in the wall of the membranous labyrinth near the sacculus.

In addition to the utriculus and the sacculus there is a third saclike structure, the *lagena*, in the membranous labyrinth of the frog. The utriculus, sacculus, and lagena each contain an ovoid cluster of calcium carbonate crystals. These three clusters are not attached to the maculae, as they are in mammals, but move freely within the endolymph. Such crystals are termed *otoliths* to distinguish them from the finely particulate otoconia typical of mammals.

The absence of the cochlea limits the frog's ability to perceive variations in tone quality. Frogs can apparently distinguish tones on the basis of pitch and intensity, but to a frog middle C probably sounds the same whether it is played on the piano, the banjo, or the trumpet.

Originally designed to effect equilibration by registering changes in the positions of otoliths, the ear has evolved into a masterpiece of mechanical engineering which registers atmospheric disturbances so slight that they cause an eardrum displacement smaller than the diameter of a molecule. During the evolution of the mammalian ear, many structures have been modified to perform new functions. The second gill-pouch wall of ancient fishes has fused with the outer skin to form the tympanum; bones which originally served as articulating portions of the upper and lower jaws have evolved into the delicate ossicles of the middle ear; the second gill pouch has become the middle-ear cavity and Eustachian tube; the perilymphatic duct, lagena, and an associated sensory area of the amphibian ear have evolved into the intricately designed mammalian cochlea; and sensory cells which originally responded only to changes in the positions of otoliths now distinguish the vast range of sounds produced by a symphony orchestra.

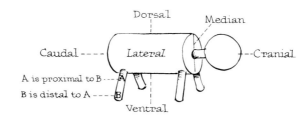

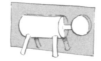

Median sagittal plane

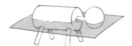

Horizontal or frontal plane

Transverse or cross plane

DEFINITIONS OF DESCRIPTIVE TERMS

Right and *left* are determined with reference to the orientation of the specimen, not with reference to the orientation of the observer.

Dorsal: toward the back, or upper side.

Ventral: toward the abdomen, or under side.

Lateral: pertaining to the side of the body.

Medial: pertaining to the middle, or midline of the body.

Distal: pertaining to a position removed from the center of the body or from the origin of a structure.

Proximal: pertaining to a position close to the center of the body or to the origin of a structure.

Anterior, cephalic or *cranial:* toward the head.

Posterior or *caudal:* toward the tail.

Deep or *central:* near the middle of the trunk or of a limb.

Superficial: near the surface of the trunk or of a limb.

Median sagittal plane: the plane which divides the body into identical halves.

Sagittal plane: any plane parallel to the median sagittal plane.

Horizontal or *frontal plane:* at right angles to the sagittal plane and parallel to the dorsal and ventral surfaces.

Transverse or *cross plane:* at right angles to both the sagittal and horizontal planes.

Bibliography

Benedict, Francis G. *Vital Energetics: A Study in Comparative Basal Metabolism.* Washington, D.C.: The Carnegie Institution, 1938.

Cowles, R. B. "Fur and Feathers—A Result of High Temperature?" *Science* (1946), 103; 2664:74-75.

———. "Evolution of Dermal Temperature Regulation," *Evolution* (1958), 12:347-57.

Crile, George. *Intelligence, Power and Personality.* New York: McGraw-Hill Book Co., Inc., 1941.

De Long, K. T. "Quantitative Analysis of Blood Circulation Through the Frog Heart," *Science*, 138 (1962), 693-94.

Hemmingsen, A. M. "The Relation of Standard (Basal) Energy Metabolism to Total Fresh Weight of Living Organisms," *Reports of the Steno Memorial Hospital (1950)*, 4:7-58.

Holmes, Samuel J. *The Biology of the Frog* (4th ed.). New York: Macmillan Co., 1934.

Hyman, Libbie H. *Comparative Vertebrate Anatomy* (2d ed.). Chicago: University of Chicago Press, 1942.

Kobler, John. *The Reluctant Surgeon.* Garden City, N.Y.: Doubleday & Co., 1960.

Moore, John A. (ed.). *Physiology of the Amphibia.* New York: Academic Press, 1964.

———. *Principles of Zoology.* New York: Oxford University Press, 1957.

Murray, Cecil D. "The Physiological Principle of Minimal Work in the Vascular System, and the Cost of Blood Volume," *Proc. Nat. Acad. Sci.*, 12 (Wash., D.C., 1926), 207-14.

Noble, G. Kingsley. *The Biology of the Amphibia.* New York: McGraw-Hill Book Co., Inc., 1931.

Prosser, C. Ladd and Frank A. Brown, Jr. *Comparative Animal Physiology* (2d ed.). Philadelphia: W. B. Saunders Co., 1961.

Romer, Alfred S. "Origin of the Amniote Egg," *Science Monthly* (1957), 85:57-63.

———. *The Vertebrate Body.* Philadelphia: W. B. Saunders Co., 1949.

Simpson, George Gaylord. *The Meaning of Evolution.* New Haven: Yale University Press, 1949.

Sisson, Septimus. *The Anatomy of Domestic Animals* (4th ed., rev. J. D. Grossman). Philadelphia: W. B. Saunders, 1953.

Smith, Hobart M. *Evolution of Chordate Structure.* New York: Holt, Rinehart & Winston, 1960.

Smith, Homer W. *From Fish to Philosopher.* New York: Doubleday & Co., 1961.

Thompson, D'Arcy Wentworth. *On Growth and Form.* New York: Macmillan Co., 1942.

Walls, Gordon Lynn. *The Vertebrate Eye and Its Adaptive Radiation.* New York: Hafner Publishing Company, 1963.

Wooldridge, Dean E. *The Machinery of the Brain.* New York: McGraw-Hill Book Co., Inc., 1963.